Discover Your Meditation

Find the Joy

Nilam Pathak

Anshuman Sharma

Aegis India PL

Contents

Dedication

To all those who would soon experience the joy of life and its every moment.

Preface

In our fast-paced, ever-changing world, finding moments of peace and clarity can seem like an elusive dream. The constant barrage of information and the demands of modern life often leave us feeling overwhelmed and disconnected from our inner selves. Meditation offers a sanctuary, a way to reconnect, find balance, and cultivate a sense of inner peace amidst the chaos. However, with the myriad of meditation techniques available, it can be daunting to know where to start or which practice might be best suited for you.

"Discover Your Meditation" is a comprehensive guide designed to demystify the world of meditation and provide you with the tools to explore and find the meditation practice that resonates most with you. Whether you are a complete beginner or an experienced practitioner looking to deepen your practice, this book aims to be your companion on this transformative journey. By providing detailed descriptions and processes for various meditation techniques, "Discover Your Meditation" aims to empower you with the knowledge and tools to embark on a transformative journey of self-discovery and inner peace.

Each chapter delves into a different meditation technique, offering clear, step-by-step instructions that you can easily follow at home. We begin with the foundational practices such as Transcendental Meditation, where the focus is on repeating a mantra to reach a state of restful alertness. You will learn how to sit comfortably, focus on your breath, and use a personal mantra to guide your mind into a peaceful state.

Next, we explore Vipassana Meditation, an ancient practice that cultivates mindfulness and insight. Through detailed guidance, you will learn how to observe your breath, bodily sensations, and thoughts without judgment, fostering a deep awareness of the present moment and the impermanent nature of all experiences.

For those who resonate with sound and music, the chapters on Sound Meditation and Music Meditation offer methods to harmonize your mind and body through auditory stimuli. You will discover how the vibrations of sound can enhance your meditative experience and lead to profound relaxation and emotional healing.

We also delve into more active forms of meditation, such as Dance Meditation and Movement Meditation, which integrate physical movement with mindfulness. These practices are perfect for those who find stillness challenging and prefer a more dynamic approach to meditation.

For a more introspective journey, Third Eye Meditation and Chakra Meditation provide techniques to tap into your inner wisdom and balance your body's energy centers. These practices can help you develop heightened intuition, spiritual awareness, and emotional stability.

Finally, we explore unique and joyful practices like Laughing Meditation and Gratitude Meditation, which focus on fostering a positive mindset and enhancing overall well-being through the simple acts of laughter and expressing gratitude.

As you journey through "Discover Your Meditation", you will not only learn about the different types of meditation but also gain insights into how each practice can benefit various aspects of your life. Our goal is to help you experiment with these techniques, find the ones that resonate with you, and incorporate them into your daily routine.

Meditation is a deeply personal journey, and what works for one person may not work for another. This book encourages you to explore, experiment, and ultimately discover the meditation practice that best suits your unique needs and preferences. May this guide serve as a beacon, illuminating your path to inner peace, clarity, and self-discovery.

Welcome to the journey of discovering your meditation.

Namaste.

Meditation- The Concept

Meditation is a practice where you focus your mind to relax, improve your concentration, or become more emotionally calm and stable. It often involves sitting quietly and paying attention to your thoughts, breath, or sensations without judgment. The goal is to clear your mind of clutter and reach a state of deeper awareness or peace, which can help reduce stress and increase overall well-being.

In the practice of meditation an individual uses techniques like mindfulness, or focusing their mind on a particular object, thought, or activity, to train attention and awareness, and achieve a mentally clear and emotionally calm and stable state. It is like giving your mind a break from being busy or stressed by concentrating on something simple and relaxing, which can help you feel more peaceful and balanced in your everyday life. The advanced practitioners of meditation can free or minimize thoughts in their minds achieving deep relaxation, experience joy, gain clarity and focus while enjoying positive effects on their body and emotions.

Meditation and Modern Life

Meditation, a practice deeply rooted in various ancient traditions, has transcended its religious and cultural origins to become a mainstream method for enhancing mental and emotional well-being.

Meditation is believed to have originated in the Eastern religious and spiritual traditions, particularly within Hinduism and Buddhism, thousands of years ago. The Vedas, ancient Hindu scriptures, mention the practice as a means to achieve spiritual enlightenment. Similarly, in Buddhism, meditation is an essential path toward awakening and understanding the nature of reality, known as Dharma. These traditional contexts view meditation as a method to transcend the mind's habitual conditioning and to uncover the innate state of peace and clarity.

Over the centuries, meditation practices have spread across the world and have been adapted and integrated into various other religions, including Christianity, Judaism, and Islam, each adding its own spiritual perspectives and practices. In these traditions, meditation is often linked with prayer, contemplation, and the seeking of a deeper relationship with the divine.

The practice of meditation reflects a deep-rooted human capacity to seek inner peace and understanding. Its enduring presence in human culture and its increasing adoption in various sectors of modern life underscore its universal appeal and applicability. Whether used for spiritual growth, health enhancement, or psychological resilience, meditation offers a profound source of calm and clarity in the complex web of modern existence. As society continues to grapple with high levels of stress and mental health challenges, meditation provides a valuable tool for individuals to regain control over their mental states and improve their quality of life.

Meditation encompasses a wide range of techniques, including mindfulness meditation, focused attention, loving-kindness meditation, and transcendental meditation, among others. These techniques vary primarily in their focus of attention and intended outcomes. Let's check some examples.

- Mindfulness meditation encourages practitioners to observe thoughts and feelings without judgment, promoting a state of awareness and presence.
- Focused attention meditation involves concentration on a single point of reference, such as the breath, a mantra, or a visual object.
- Loving-kindness meditation (Metta) aims to cultivate an attitude of love and kindness towards everything, even sources of stress and the individuals we perceive as enemies.

- Transcendental Meditation uses a mantra or a repetitive sound to help the mind settle into a state of profound rest and relaxation.

Scientific research has validated many health benefits of meditation, revealing its significant impact on both the mind and body. Physiologically, meditation has been shown to reduce stress, control anxiety, improve cardiovascular health, and enhance overall well-being. It achieves this by altering the body's stress response via decreased cortisol production and sympathetic nervous system activity.

Psychologically, meditation helps enhance self-awareness, reduces negative emotions, increases imagination and creativity, and improves patience and tolerance. Neuroscientific studies have demonstrated that regular meditation can lead to neuroplasticity, where the brain undergoes changes in structure and function, particularly in areas associated with memory, self-awareness, and empathy.

In today's fast-paced world, the calming effects of meditation are perhaps more relevant than ever. With the rise of digital technology and social media, individuals face constant distractions and overstimulation, making the focused, quiet practice of meditation an effective counterbalance. Many people turn to meditation as a tool for mental health management, to improve concentration, and to maintain emotional balance amidst the stresses of daily life.

Furthermore, meditation has been integrated into various health and wellness programs. It is frequently used in clinical settings as part of psychotherapy, particularly in Cognitive Behavioral Therapy (CBT) and mindfulness-based stress reduction (MBSR) programs. Schools, workplaces, and even prisons have adopted meditation programs to reduce stress and improve emotional well-being.

The Discovery of Meditation

Meditation has gained significant traction as a beneficial practice for mental and physical health, with a wide array of studies backing its positive impacts.

Popularity and Demographics: Meditation is practiced by a broad range of individuals globally. In the United States, meditation has seen a sharp increase in popularity, especially among adults aged 45-64, who are the most likely to meditate. Additionally, women are more likely to engage in meditation than men. According to Pew Research, 55% of women and 45% of men meditate at least once a week.

Meditation in Schools and Workplaces: Meditation is increasingly being incorporated into educational and professional settings due to its benefits in reducing stress and improving focus and productivity. For instance, some schools have reported a reduction in suspensions and improvements in student behavior and sleep after introducing meditation programs. Similarly, many companies have started offering meditation programs, noting significant improvements in employee productivity and a decrease in absenteeism.

Health Benefits: Meditation has been shown to offer numerous health benefits. According to researchers, meditation can reduce symptoms of anxiety by 60% after 6-9 months of practice and can decrease depression relapses by up to 12%. Meditation also significantly lowers blood pressure in hypertensive patients.

Mental and Cognitive Improvements: Short-term practice of mindfulness meditation can enhance attention span and visuospatial processing in just four days. Long-term practice can increase gray matter density in the brain, particularly in areas associated with memory, learning, and emotional regulation.

Brain Function: Recent studies have shown that meditation can significantly enhance brain function. For example, just 8 weeks of meditation training can lead to faster switching between different states of consciousness, enhancing the brain's ability to maintain focus and attention.

Advanced Meditation Techniques: Advanced forms of meditation have been shown to impact various areas of the brain including the cortex, subcortex, brainstem, and cerebellum. This not only affects attention and self-perception but also equips the brain with the ability to handle various mental health conditions more effectively.

Mental Health: Meditation is effective in treating anxiety, depression, and stress, with numerous studies reporting positive outcomes. It's also used in enhancing levels of mindfulness and improving mental disorders in both adults and children.

Physical Health: Beyond mental health, meditation also offers physical health benefits. It has been found to help with high blood pressure, stress related symptoms, and chronic pain. Meditation not only alleviates physical symptoms but also enhances overall vitality and quality of life.

The scientific community continues to explore meditation through advanced imaging and other research techniques. This research aims to bridge the gap between traditional meditative practices and contemporary clinical practices, potentially leading to innovative treatments for mental health conditions and improving societal well-being.

The Need for Meditation

The integration of meditation into daily life can offer profound benefits across many aspects of health and well-being. Whether coping with stress, improving physical health, or enhancing mental and emotional resilience, meditation provides tools that can help individuals manage their lives more effectively. These benefits make meditation a valuable practice for people of all ages and backgrounds, contributing to a more balanced and fulfilling life.

Meditation is increasingly recognized for its wide-ranging benefits, making it a valuable practice for many people. Following are some key reasons to understand the importance of meditation:

<u>Stress Reduction</u>: Meditation is perhaps most sought out for its ability to reduce stress. Techniques like mindfulness meditation help lower levels of cortisol, the stress hormone, thereby alleviating stress symptoms.

<u>Enhances Emotional Health</u>: Regular meditation can lead to an improved self-image and a more positive outlook on life. Certain forms of meditation, such as mindfulness, can decrease levels of depression and anxiety.

Improves Concentration: Meditation has been shown to help increase the strength and endurance of your attention. Regular practice can help increase focus, even in children, and enhance the ability to perform under pressure.

Promotes General Well-being: Many people report feeling greater peace and happiness as they incorporate meditation into their daily lives. This sense of well-being can be attributed to meditation's effect on the brain and emotional response handling.

Physical Health Benefits: Meditation practices can also lead to physical health benefits such as improved blood pressure, reduced chronic pain, and alleviation of gastrointestinal difficulties. It can also enhance the immune system and help fight diseases.

Helps with Sleep: Insomnia and other sleep issues can often be improved through meditation, which helps in relaxing the mind and body, making it easier to fall asleep and stay asleep.

Cognitive and Neurological Benefits: Studies have shown that meditation can thicken the prefrontal cortex and increase gray matter in the brain, which are associated with higher-order brain functions like awareness, concentration, and decision-making.

Emotional Resilience: By enabling better control over processing feelings and emotions, meditation can contribute to greater resilience against emotional stress.

Slows Aging: Some research suggests that meditation can influence telomere length, an essential part of human cells that affect how our cells age, potentially slowing the aging process at a cellular level.

Improvement in Relationships: Meditation can enhance emotional intelligence and the capacity to relate to others. By improving your awareness and empathy, it can lead to healthier and more fulfilling relationships. This aspect is especially beneficial in resolving conflicts and understanding others better.

Reduction in Memory Loss: Meditation, particularly techniques that emphasize concentration and memory training, can help in the fight against age-related memory loss and dementia. It has been shown to improve short and long-term recall in both young adults and the elderly.

Management of Addiction: The self-control developed through meditation can help people recover from addiction by increasing their awareness of triggers for addictive behaviors. Mindfulness training is an integral part of many substance abuse programs because it teaches patients to redirect their attention, manage their emotions, and improve their overall psychological well-being.

Enhanced Self-Awareness: Some forms of meditation can help you develop a stronger understanding of yourself, helping you grow into your best self. By building greater self-awareness and self-esteem, meditation can help people steer away from negative patterns of thought and replace them with positive ones.

Healthy Heart: Meditation has cardiovascular benefits as well. It can help in controlling blood pressure by reducing stress and enabling the body to relax. This decrease in blood pressure can lower the risk of heart disease and stroke.

Pain Management: Studies have shown that meditation can reduce the perception of pain in the brain. This can help chronic pain sufferers feel less pain and, in some cases, lessen their dependence on pain medications.

This is not Meditation

Several practices are often confused with meditation, but they differ in intent, focus, or methodology. Each of these activities has its own value and place but should not be confused with meditation, which is a specific practice aimed at developing mindfulness, concentration, and deeper self-awareness. There could be some overlapping aspects of these activities with meditation which could be the starting steps for meditation. Any activity that can give the control of your thoughts and mind can be a supporting element for meditation.

Understanding these distinctions helps clarify the unique characteristics of meditation, emphasizing its role in fostering deep awareness, mental clarity, and a state of mindful presence that is distinct from simply relaxing or engaging in other mentally or physically intensive activities.

Deep Relaxation or Sleep: While meditation involves a level of relaxation, it's fundamentally an alert, aware state. Some might think lying down and letting the mind drift off (as in sleep or daydreaming) is meditation. However, the goal of meditation is to remain aware and focused, rather than drifting into unconsciousness.

Hypnosis: Hypnosis and meditation both involve altered states of consciousness, but they serve different purposes. Hypnosis is usually directed by another person and aims to induce a highly suggestible state for therapeutic purposes. In contrast, meditation is typically self-directed and focuses on self-awareness and the present moment.

Mind Wandering: Sometimes people confuse meditation with the act of letting the mind wander freely. While meditation might involve observation of thoughts, it's about doing so with detachment and focus, rather than getting lost in the thoughts themselves.

Simple Relaxation Activities: Activities like listening to music, taking a bath, or walking can be relaxing and therapeutic but are not meditation. Meditation requires a deliberate focus on a particular object, thought, activity, or nothing at all, with the intent of increasing awareness of the present.

Prayer: While prayer and meditation can look similar externally, prayer typically involves speaking to or asking for assistance from a deity or external force, often with a focus on something other than oneself. Meditation tends to focus inward on the self, breath, or consciousness.

Focused Work or Study: Engaging deeply in activities such as reading, writing, or artistic creation involves concentration but is not meditation. These activities are goal-directed and involve active mental engagement with content, whereas meditation generally aims to transcend such engagements and often seeks to quieten the mind.

Physical Exercise: Although activities like yoga or tai chi incorporate mindfulness and can be meditative, traditional physical exercise itself (like running or lifting weights) is not meditation. These activities can be performed meditatively but their primary focus is on physical exertion and fitness, not the cultivation of mindfulness or inner silence.

Positive Thinking or Visualization: These practices involve consciously directing thoughts towards positive outcomes or visualizing success and happiness. While they may incorporate elements of focus similar to meditation, they are goal-oriented and involve active mental engagement, aiming at influencing real-world outcomes, rather than observing thoughts without attachment as in meditation.

Stress Management Techniques: Techniques like deep breathing exercises or progressive muscle relaxation are often used to manage stress and can be components of a meditation practice, but on their own, they do not constitute the full scope of meditation. These practices are usually more focused on physical relaxation rather than cultivating a deep, ongoing state of mental awareness.

Leisure Activities: Engaging in hobbies or leisure activities such as gardening, painting, or cooking is therapeutic and can be quite absorbing but isn't meditation. Although these activities can be performed mindfully and help one achieve a flow state, meditation is distinct in its systematic approach to developing detachment from moment-to-moment thoughts and deepening awareness of the mind-body connection.

Basic Process of Meditation

Meditation is a practice where an individual uses a technique, such as mindfulness, or focusing the mind on a particular object, thought, or activity, to train attention and awareness, and achieve a mentally clear and emotionally calm and stable state.

The Process:

1. Choose a Quiet Location: Find a quiet place free from distractions. This helps in maintaining focus and minimizes external disturbances.
2. Set a Time Limit: Especially for beginners, starting with short periods of meditation, such as 5-10 minutes, is beneficial. As one becomes more comfortable with the process, the duration can be gradually increased.
3. Adopt a Comfortable Posture: You can sit on a chair, a cushion, or a meditation bench. The important thing is to keep your back upright in a

comfortable position. This posture aids in staying alert and focused during the session.

4. Close Your Eyes: This helps in reducing external visual distractions and makes it easier to focus internally.
5. Breathe Naturally: Pay attention to the natural inhalation and exhalation of your breath. Feel the breath as it enters and leaves your nostrils or notice your belly rising and falling.
6. Focus Your Attention: As you meditate, you will notice your mind wandering. When you realize that your thoughts have drifted, gently redirect your focus back to your breath or chosen object of meditation without judgment.
7. End the Session Slowly: When you are ready to end your session, open your eyes and slowly acclimatize yourself back to your surroundings. Take a moment to notice any sounds in the environment, how your body feels, your thoughts, and emotions.

Start your journey of meditation with this simple process.

Meditation Transformation

Practicing meditation regularly exhibits several distinct characteristics and traits that reflect the deep impacts of this practice on both the mind and body.

These characteristics combine to form a profile of an individual who is not only mentally and physically healthier but also more content and fulfilled in their daily life. It shapes not just the mind and body, but also deeply influences personal habits, social interactions, and overall approach to life. The transformative effects of meditation are profound and wide-reaching, impacting virtually every aspect of a practitioner's existence.

Let's understand the profile of such an individual:

Increased Emotional Stability: Long-term meditators often show greater emotional resilience, meaning they manage stress and recover from negative emotional events more effectively. This is partly due to enhanced regulation of the amygdala, the brain's response center for emotions, particularly fear and stress reactions.

Enhanced Concentration and Attention: Regular meditation is associated with improved attention, concentration, and the ability to keep the mind steady and focused. Studies have shown that meditation can thicken the prefrontal cortex, which governs these abilities.

Reduced Aging Effects on the Brain: Meditation can also slow some of the natural age-related decline in brain structure and function. Long-term meditators often have better-preserved brains as they age, with more grey matter volume and density.

Heightened Self-Awareness: Individuals who have meditated for years tend to have a heightened sense of self-awareness. This is due to the introspective nature of meditation, which enhances one's ability to examine thoughts and emotions objectively.

Greater Compassion and Empathy: Meditation practices like loving-kindness (Metta) enhance feelings of compassion and empathy toward others. This could be due to changes in brain areas related to empathy and emotional processing.

Improved Physical Health: Long-term meditation is correlated with better physical health, including lower blood pressure, reduced chronic pain, and an enhanced immune system. These benefits arise from reduced stress levels and a healthier lifestyle that often accompanies regular meditation practice.

Mindfulness in Daily Life: Long-term meditators often carry mindfulness into their daily activities. This means they are generally more present, attentive, and aware throughout the day, which enhances the quality of their interactions and tasks.

Spiritual Fulfillment: For many, prolonged meditation deepens spiritual life, providing a sense of peace, connectedness, and fulfillment that permeates their existence.

Lifestyle Choices: Meditators often embrace healthier lifestyles, including diet, exercise, and abstaining from harmful habits like smoking or excessive drinking. This is partly due to increased self-awareness and the desire to maintain the clarity and calm achieved through meditation.

Cognitive Flexibility: They typically exhibit greater cognitive flexibility, enabling them to adapt to new situations and think outside the box. This is linked to the brain's enhanced ability to reorganize itself by forming new neural connections.

Reduced Reactivity: Individuals who engage in long-term meditation often display less emotional reactivity. They are better able to handle stress without reacting impulsively, which reflects enhanced emotional regulation skills fostered by consistent meditation practice.

Improved Relationships: With increased empathy, emotional stability, and reduced reactivity, long-term meditators often enjoy stronger and more harmonious relationships. Their ability to listen actively and respond thoughtfully can lead to deeper connections with others.

Deep Sleep: Regular meditation is associated with improved quality of sleep. Long-term practitioners often report deeper sleep and feel more rested. This is partly due to the calming effects of meditation on the mind, which facilitates easier transitions into deep sleep.

Enhanced Problem-Solving Skills: Meditation enhances the ability to detach from immediate emotional responses and view problems more dispassionately. This detachment allows for clearer thinking and better decision-making, which are valuable in personal and professional contexts.

Cultural and Ethical Sensitivity: Meditation often involves elements of ethical training, introspection, and the cultivation of virtues. As a result, long-term practitioners may develop a heightened sense of ethical responsibility and cultural sensitivity.

Reduced Dependence on External Sources of Happiness: Long-term meditators often find joy and satisfaction from within rather than relying heavily on external circumstances or material possessions. This internal source of happiness contributes to a more stable and sustained sense of well-being.

Neurological Health: Studies suggest that meditation can help prevent neurodegenerative diseases or mitigate their effects. The practice is associated with increased levels of brain-derived neurotrophic factor (BDNF), a protein that supports brain health.

Heightened Intuition: Many meditators report an enhanced sense of intuition, likely due to greater attunement with their internal mental and emotional states. This intuition can manifest as a better understanding of personal needs and the intentions of others.

Greater Overall Contentment: The combination of physical health, emotional stability, and mental clarity often leads to a profound sense of overall contentment in life. Long-term meditators frequently report higher life satisfaction and a greater sense of fulfillment.

Meditation Basics

Meditation involves a set of foundational practices that help establish and maintain a disciplined meditation routine. Following are the fundamentals that are often emphasized across various forms of meditation:

Setting and Environment: A calm and quiet environment is crucial for meditation. This helps minimize distractions and facilitates deeper focus and relaxation. Comfortable settings can vary from a specific room in a house to any quiet spot where regular practice can be maintained.

Posture: Proper posture is essential, whether sitting on a chair, cushion, or mat. The spine should be upright but not stiff, with hands resting comfortably on the knees or in the lap. This posture helps maintain alertness and allows for effective breathing.

Breath Focus: Many meditation techniques emphasize focusing on the breath. This involves observing the natural inhalation and exhalation without trying to control it. Breath focus is a tool to anchor the mind and cultivate mindfulness or concentration.

Attention and Concentration: The core of meditation is the practice of directing and sustaining attention. Whether focusing on the breath, a mantra, a visual object, or even an idea, the ability to keep the mind steady on one point is fundamental. When distractions occur, the practice involves gently returning the focus to the chosen object of meditation.

Mindfulness: This involves being present and fully engaged with whatever activity one is doing, free from distraction or judgment. Mindfulness can be practiced during meditation by observing thoughts, feelings, and sensations as they arise and pass, without becoming involved with them.

Regular Practice: Consistency is key in meditation. Regular practice helps to develop the skills and benefits of meditation more deeply. Setting a specific time and duration for daily practice can aid in developing a routine.

Attitude and Approach: An open, patient, and non-judgmental attitude is essential when meditating. Meditation is not about achieving immediate results but about ongoing practice and experiencing whatever arises with acceptance.

Progressive Relaxation: Some meditation practices involve progressively relaxing different parts of the body. This helps reduce physical tension and facilitates mental relaxation, allowing for a deeper meditative state.

Ending the Session: Concluding a meditation session gently is important. Taking a few moments to transition out of meditation can help carry the calmness and mindfulness into everyday activities.

Reflection and Application: After meditation, reflecting on the experience and applying insights gained during practice to everyday life can enhance the benefits of meditation, making it a transformative tool for personal growth.

Integration into Daily Life: For meditation to be most effective, it's beneficial to integrate the qualities and awareness developed during meditation into daily activities. This might involve practicing mindfulness during routine tasks like eating, walking, or interacting with others, thereby cultivating a continuous state of presence and attentiveness.

Use of Mantras: In some meditation traditions, particularly in Transcendental Meditation, mantras are used as the focal point of practice. A mantra is a sound, word, or phrase repeated to aid concentration in meditation. It helps keep the mind focused and can elevate the meditator's state of consciousness.

Visualization: Some meditation techniques involve visualization to focus the mind or cultivate certain qualities such as peace or compassion. This could involve picturing a peaceful scene, visualizing light or energy, or imagining the self as embodying these qualities.

Cultivation of Specific Qualities: Certain forms of meditation specifically aim to develop qualities such as compassion, loving-kindness, patience, and gratitude.

For example, Metta or loving-kindness meditation involves mentally sending goodwill and kindness to oneself and others.

Silence and Stillness: Embracing silence and stillness is a fundamental aspect of many meditative practices. It involves quieting the mind and finding tranquility and peace within, which helps deepen the meditation experience.

Dealing with Distractions: Learning how to handle distractions is a crucial part of meditation. This involves recognizing when the mind has wandered and gently bringing it back to the focus of meditation without criticism or frustration.

Guided Meditation: For beginners, guided meditations can be very helpful. These are typically led by an experienced practitioner either in person or via a recording. The guidance can help newcomers understand what to do and how to handle common challenges in meditation.

Mindful Movement: Practices like yoga, tai chi, or qigong combine meditation with movement. These practices emphasize mindful movement and breathing to support physical health and mental clarity.

Meditation Principles

The principles of meditation often revolve around a set of core concepts that guide the practice, regardless of the specific meditation technique being used.

These principles help shape the meditation experience, making it more effective and meaningful. They are designed to cultivate a peaceful mind, enhanced awareness, and deeper understanding, all of which contribute to greater overall well-being. The specified principles not only enrich the practice itself but also enhance the overall quality of life, making meditation a transformative and integral part of daily living. Each principle supports the others, creating a comprehensive framework that fosters deep personal growth and well-being. Every principle contributes to a holistic approach to meditation, emphasizing that it is not just a practice but a way of living that influences every aspect of life. By embracing these principles, individuals can ensure their meditation practice is balanced, deeply transformative, and sustainable.

Here are some of the fundamental principles:

Principle of Consistency: Regular practice is crucial in meditation. Consistent practice helps to deepen the meditative state and makes it easier to access that state of mind during everyday activities.

Principle of Patience: Meditation requires patience both in terms of immediate practice and long-term benefits. Changes and benefits can be subtle and gradual, so being patient is essential for developing a lasting and effective meditation routine.

Principle of Non-judgment: One of the key principles in meditation is to observe thoughts, sensations, and emotions without judgment. This means letting go of evaluation and criticism and simply witnessing the mind's activity as it unfolds.

Principle of Beginner's Mind: Approaching meditation with a beginner's mind, regardless of experience level, involves being open to each experience as if it were the first. This attitude encourages openness and curiosity in practice.

Principle of Letting Go: A crucial aspect of meditation is the ability to let go of attachment, thoughts, narratives, and outcomes. This involves releasing the need to control the experience and allowing the practice to flow naturally.

Principle of Mindfulness: Staying present during meditation practice is essential. Mindfulness is about being fully engaged in the here and now, paying attention to the present moment without distraction or dwelling on the past or future.

Principle of Focus and Concentration: Many forms of meditation involve concentration on a particular object, thought, or activity, such as the breath, a mantra, or a visual object. Developing focus is key to managing the mind's tendency to wander.

Principle of Acceptance: Part of meditation is learning to accept whatever arises. This includes accepting feelings, thoughts, and bodily sensations without trying to change them.

Principle of Compassion: In meditation, especially in practices like Metta or loving-kindness meditation, there is an emphasis on developing compassion towards oneself and others. This fosters a sense of connectedness and empathy.

Principle of Balance: Meditation often seeks to find a balance between effort and ease. Too much effort can lead to tension and frustration, while too little can lead to sluggishness or lack of focus.

Principle of Simplicity: Keeping the meditation practice simple is key, especially for beginners. Overcomplicating the process with too many techniques or expectations can hinder progress. Focus on one technique that resonates and stick with it.

Principle of Intention: Setting a clear intention before beginning a meditation session can guide your practice.

It helps direct your energy and attention and defines what you wish to achieve or cultivate, such as calmness, relaxation, or insight.

Principle of Silence: Embracing silence is an essential part of deepening the meditative experience. Silence isn't just a lack of external noise; it also involves quieting the inner chatter of the mind to foster a greater sense of peace.

Principle of Respect for the Process: Respect for the practice of meditation and the journey it entails is crucial. This involves recognizing that each session is a step towards greater self-awareness and self-mastery.

Principle of Commitment: Meditation requires a commitment to practice regularly and to engage with the process, even when it feels challenging or when life becomes busy. This commitment is crucial for experiencing the profound benefits of meditation.

Principle of Holistic Integration: Integrating the insights and calmness gained from meditation into daily life is one of the ultimate goals of the practice. It's about bringing the peace and balance experienced during meditation into interactions and activities throughout the day.

Principle of Ethical Living: Many meditation traditions emphasize the importance of ethical conduct as foundational to effective practice. This includes principles such as non-harming, truthfulness, and generosity, which support a clear conscience and reduce internal conflict.

Principle of Adaptability: Flexibility in meditation practice can be essential, especially as one progresses or as life circumstances change. Adapting the practice to meet current physical, emotional, or time constraints while maintaining the essence of meditation can help sustain a regular practice over time.

Principle of Non-attachment: This principle involves not clinging to specific outcomes or experiences during meditation. By practicing non-attachment, meditators learn to appreciate the process without becoming frustrated by the lack of perceived progress or specific results. It encourages openness to whatever arises during meditation.

Principle of Energy Management: Understanding and managing one's energy through meditation can enhance the practice. This can involve recognizing when energy levels are low and perhaps opting for more gentle or restorative practices or harnessing higher energy for more focused forms of meditation.

Principle of Equanimity: Developing equanimity through meditation involves maintaining mental calmness, composure, and evenness of temper, especially in difficult situations. This quality helps meditators remain steady with a sense of inner peace, regardless of the external circumstances.

Principle of Mind-Body Connection: Acknowledging and nurturing the connection between the mind and body is a crucial meditation principle. Techniques that enhance this awareness, like mindful breathing or body scan meditations, help to integrate and harmonize physical sensations with mental states.

Principle of Gratitude: Cultivating gratitude as part of meditation practice can shift the focus from what is lacking to appreciating what is present. This shift in perspective can significantly enhance psychological resilience and contentment.

Principle of Continuous Learning: The journey of meditation is one of continuous learning and discovery. Engaging with new teachings, refining techniques, and staying open to insights not only enrich the practice but also fuel personal growth and understanding.

Need for Meditation Discovery

The journey of discovering the meditation process most suitable for you is illuminating and rewarding. You may need to understand and try few techniques to experience their impact and effectiveness. By experimenting with different types of meditation, you can discover which practice feels most natural and beneficial, thereby enhancing your overall well-being and making meditation an enjoyable, rewarding, and integral part of your daily routine. Discovering the type of meditation that is most effective for you is crucial for several reasons, with an objective to a more satisfying and beneficial practice.

<u>Personal Compatibility</u>: Meditation comes in many forms, each with unique focuses and techniques, such as mindfulness, transcendental, guided visualization, or loving-kindness meditation. Finding a method that resonates with your personal preferences, beliefs, and psychological needs can significantly enhance your engagement and the likelihood of maintaining a consistent practice.

<u>Specific Benefits</u>: Different types of meditation offer specific benefits. For instance, mindfulness meditation is known for enhancing awareness and reducing stress,

while loving-kindness meditation may be more effective at fostering empathy and positive emotions towards oneself and others. Identifying your personal goals and needs can help you choose a meditation style that best addresses them.

Cognitive Styles: People have different cognitive styles, some may find focusing on a mantra helpful, while others may prefer a more open monitoring style, like mindfulness. Identifying a meditation practice that aligns with your natural thinking pattern can make the practice more intuitive and effective.

Physical and Emotional Needs: Depending on your physical and emotional state, certain practices might be more beneficial than others. For example, someone dealing with depression may find mindfulness or compassion-focused meditations particularly therapeutic, whereas someone looking to enhance concentration might benefit from focused attention meditation.

Sustainability of Practice: When you find a meditation style that suits you, you are more likely to stick with it long-term. Regular and sustained practice is key to reaping the profound benefits of meditation, including enhanced mental, emotional, and physical health.

Adaptation to Lifestyle: Your lifestyle can also dictate the most suitable type of meditation. Busy individuals might prefer shorter, more flexible practices like mindful breathing during breaks, whereas others might have the time and inclination for longer sessions involving guided meditations.

Enhanced Progress and Development: When a meditation practice aligns well with your personal characteristics and life circumstances, you are more likely to experience rapid and profound progress. This compatibility can accelerate your development in areas such as self-awareness, emotional regulation, and cognitive resilience.

Deeper Insights: Practicing the right type of meditation for your needs and personality can lead to deeper insights into your behavior, thoughts, and emotions. This can enhance personal growth and lead to significant life changes and improvements.

Avoidance of Negative Experiences: Not all meditation techniques are suitable for everyone, and some can even provoke anxiety or increase mental distress in certain individuals. For example, intense concentration practices might be overwhelming for some, while open awareness practices might be too unstructured for others. Finding a method that feels comfortable and safe can help avoid these negative experiences.

Customization and Adaptability: As you grow and change, your meditation needs may evolve. Starting with a practice that suits you can provide a solid foundation for adapting or expanding your practice to include other forms of meditation as your interests and needs develop.

Maximizing Time and Effort: Given the investment of time and effort required to maintain a meditation practice, it's practical to choose a method that provides the most benefits and enjoyment. This ensures that the time you dedicate to meditation is used effectively, giving you the greatest return on your investment.

Discover your Meditation

Discovering the type of meditation that best suits you involves exploring various practices to find one that aligns with your personal preferences, goals, and lifestyle. This personal alignment is crucial because it enhances the effectiveness, enjoyment, and sustainability of the practice, making it a more integral and beneficial part of your daily life.

The endeavor to discover your meditation is a personal process that can profoundly affect your well-being and quality of life. It requires patience, openness, and a willingness to explore and engage with different practices. By finding a meditation style that you can connect with deeply, you set the foundation for a sustained and fulfilling practice.

Finding the right type of meditation is a journey of exploration and experimentation.

The Process

Research Different Types: Start by gaining an understanding of the various types of meditation available. Some popular forms include mindfulness meditation, transcendental meditation, guided visualization, loving-kindness meditation, and focused attention meditation. Researching these can help you understand their distinct methods and benefits.

Identify Your Goals: Reflect on what you hope to achieve through meditation. Are you looking for stress reduction, increased focus, emotional healing, spiritual growth, or perhaps a combination of these? Different techniques have different strengths and knowing your goals can help narrow down the options.

Experiment with Techniques: Try out several types of meditation to see which one resonates with you. Many community centers, wellness programs, and apps offer introductory sessions that can give you a taste of various practices. Commit to each type for a short period, such as a week or two, to truly experience its impact.

Assess Your Comfort and Response: As you try different types, pay attention to how you feel during and after the sessions. Do you feel more relaxed, agitated, clear-headed, or confused? Your body's and mind's responses can be great indicators of whether a particular style is suitable for you.

Seek Guidance: Consider taking a class or finding a meditation teacher. A knowledgeable guide can provide valuable insights into different practices and offer suggestions based on your individual needs and temperament.

Evaluate Your Progress: After experimenting with various forms, evaluate which practice has brought you the most personal satisfaction and improvement in the areas you are focusing on. Consider factors like ease of practice, immediate feelings of well-being, and long-term benefits.

Refine Your Practice: Once you find a method that seems like a good fit, continue to refine your practice. As you grow and your life changes, you might need to adjust your meditation practice or possibly incorporate additional practices.

Integrate into Daily Life: Finally, look for ways to integrate the benefits of your chosen meditation into your daily life. This might mean setting a regular schedule for practice, using brief mindfulness exercises during breaks at work, or applying meditative principles to interactions with others.

Maintain Flexibility and Openness: As you progress in your meditation journey, maintain flexibility and openness to changes in your practice. What works for you at one stage of your life may not be as effective at another. Be willing to reassess and adjust your practice as needed based on evolving goals, life circumstances, and personal growth.

Keep a Meditation Journal: Keeping a meditation journal can be a valuable tool. Document your experiences, feelings, and any insights that arise during and after each meditation session. This can help you track your progress, understand your reactions, and make more informed decisions about which types of meditation are most beneficial for you.

Engage with a Community: Engaging with a community of meditators can provide support, deepen your practice, and offer new perspectives. Whether it's through online forums, local meditation groups, or workshops, being part of a community can enhance your motivation and commitment to meditation.

Regular Assessments: Periodically assess the impact of your meditation practice on your overall well-being. Consider how it affects your stress levels, emotional state, mental clarity, and physical health. This ongoing evaluation can guide you in fine-tuning your practice to better meet your needs.

Incorporate Mindfulness into Everyday Activities: Try to extend the awareness and calmness you cultivate during meditation into your daily activities. Practice being present and mindful during routine tasks such as eating, walking, or even during conversations. This helps solidify meditation as not just a practice, but a way of living.

Seek Continuous Learning: The field of meditation is vast and rich with various traditions, techniques, and teachings. Continue learning about meditation through books, workshops, retreats, and courses. This will not only keep your practice vibrant but also ensure you are well-informed about the nuances and deeper aspects of meditation.

Practice Patience and Compassion: Finally, practice patience and compassion with yourself as you explore and grow in your meditation practice. Some days might be challenging, and progress might seem slow at times. Treat yourself with kindness and remember that the journey itself is just as important as the destination.

Follow these steps to discover and nurture a meditation practice that resonates deeply with you and enriches your life. Remember, the goal of meditation is not perfection but progress and personal growth.

Types of Meditation

This segment will discuss most effective meditation practices with the summary of the idea, logic and the indicative process to experience its impact.

Mindfulness Meditation

Mindful meditation, often referred to simply as mindfulness, is a form of meditation rooted in Buddhist tradition. The core concept of mindfulness is the practice of maintaining a moment-by-moment awareness of our thoughts, feelings, bodily sensations, and the surrounding environment with openness, curiosity, and non-judgment.

Mindfulness meditation encourages the practitioner to observe wandering thoughts as they drift through the mind. The intention is not to get involved with the thoughts or to judge them, but simply to be aware of each mental note as it arises. Through mindfulness meditation, you can see how your thoughts and feelings tend to move in particular patterns. Over time, you can become more aware of the human tendency to quickly judge an experience as good or bad, pleasant, or unpleasant. With practice, an inner balance develops.

Indicative Process of Mindful Meditation

The practice of mindful meditation involves several steps:

1. Find a Quiet Space: Choose a quiet and calm environment where you can relax without interruption. This can be anywhere that you find peaceful, such as a corner of your bedroom, a secluded spot in your garden, or anywhere you can sit comfortably without being disturbed.
2. Set a Time Limit: If you're just beginning, it might help to choose a short time, such as five or ten minutes. As you get more used to meditation, you can gradually extend your meditation time.
3. Assume a Comfortable Posture: You can sit on a chair with your feet on the floor, on a cushion on the floor, or in any seated comfortable position. It's important to keep your back erect but not too tight; hands on your knees or lap; shoulders and neck relaxed, and your eyes can be open or closed.
4. Focus on Your Breath: Turn your attention to the breath, a common anchor of mindfulness meditation. Notice the sensation of air entering your nostrils and leaving your mouth, or your belly rising and falling as you inhale and exhale. You don't need to control the breath, just observe it.
5. Return to the Breath When Distracted: No matter how many times you lose focus, simply return your attention back to your breath. You might find yourself distracted by noises, wandering

thoughts, or bodily sensations. When you notice this happening, gently bring your attention back to your breathing.

6. Observe Without Judgment: Try to adopt an attitude of open curiosity about your thoughts and sensations. Instead of labeling them as good or bad, or getting caught up in their content, simply note them and let them go.
7. End with Kindness: When you are ready, gently lift your gaze (if your eyes were closed) and take a moment to notice any sounds in the environment. Notice how your body feels right now. Notice your thoughts and emotions. Finishing with a moment of gratitude can enhance the benefits of your practice.

Mindful meditation can be practiced at any time of the day, integrating mindfulness into your daily routine. Over time, this form of meditation can help you develop a greater awareness of the unity of mind and body, as well as a deeper understanding of how your thoughts and feelings can impact your health and quality of life.

Transcendental Meditation

Transcendental Meditation (TM) is a form of silent mantra meditation, developed by Maharishi Mahesh Yogi. It gained popularity in the 1960s and 70s, becoming one of the most recognized and practiced forms of meditation around the world. The core idea of TM is to allow your mind to settle inward beyond thought to experience the source of thought, pure awareness or transcendental consciousness. This state of consciousness is said to be a state of profound stillness that underlies all mental activity.

Characteristics of Transcendental Meditation:

Mantra-based: TM involves the use of a specific and personalized mantra given by a certified teacher. The mantra, which is a sound or vibration, is used silently as a tool to help settle the mind.

Effortless: One of the primary principles of TM is its effortlessness. Unlike other forms of meditation that involve concentration or contemplation, TM is practiced by allowing the mind to naturally transcend the process of thought.

Non-secular: Although its origins are rooted in the Vedic tradition of India, TM is taught in a secular context, making it accessible to the whole world, irrespective of any differences.

Indicative Process of Transcendental Meditation

Transcendental Meditation (TM) is a simple and natural technique practiced for 20 minutes twice a day while sitting comfortably with your eyes closed. This is an indicative process to practice Transcendental Meditation:

1. Find a Quiet Space: Choose a comfortable, quiet place where you can sit without being disturbed.
2. Sit Comfortably: Sit in a comfortable chair with your feet on the ground and your hands on your lap. Ensure you're sitting upright but not stiff.
3. Close Your Eyes: Close your eyes and take a few deep breaths to relax. Keep your eyes closed throughout the meditation.
4. Repeat a Mantra: Silently start repeating a mantra. In TM, mantras are typically provided by certified teachers, but a simple sound like "Om" or "Ah" can be used if you don't have an official TM mantra. The mantra is a consistent rhythmic

sound without any meaning used to help your mind settle down.

5. Let the Mantra Flow: Don't concentrate or force the mantra. Let it come naturally and softly. If your mind wanders, gently bring your attention back to the mantra.
6. Continue for 20 Minutes: Keep meditating for about 20 minutes. If you lose track of the mantra, it is fine. Just come back to it gently when you realize you are off track. You can set a gentle alarm to signal the end of your meditation period.
7. Gradually End the Session: After 20 minutes, stop repeating the mantra and sit quietly with your eyes closed for a few more minutes. This allows you to transition back to your normal state of awareness smoothly.
8. Open Your Eyes: After a few minutes of sitting quietly, slowly open your eyes. Take a moment before you get up to fully return to your normal activities.

Make it Effective

- Regular Practice: Consistency is key. Try to practice TM twice a day, once in the morning and once in the evening.
- Comfort: Make sure you're physically comfortable to avoid distractions during meditation.

- Non-judgmental Awareness: If thoughts come up during meditation, don't judge them or yourself. Simply return to your mantra.

Transcendental Meditation is a straightforward practice that can be done by anyone, anywhere. By dedicating just 20 minutes twice a day, you can experience profound benefits such as reduced stress, increased relaxation, and enhanced overall well-being.

The uniqueness of TM lies in its simplicity and depth. By regularly practicing TM, individuals often report reduced stress and anxiety, improved focus and creativity, and overall greater well-being. It's recommended to learn TM from a certified teacher to ensure the authenticity of the practice and the correct usage of the mantra.

For personalized guidance and to learn the official TM technique and mantra, consider reaching out to a certified Transcendental Meditation teacher.

Guided Meditation

Guided meditation, as the name suggests, involves meditating with the guidance of a narrator or instructor who leads the session. This type of meditation is particularly useful for beginners or those who prefer structured meditation sessions. The guide provides step-by-step instructions on what to focus on and how to direct one's thoughts, often leading the practitioner through a series of mental images or scenarios designed to induce relaxation, mindfulness, or focus on specific goals like stress reduction or healing.

Characteristics of Guided Meditation

Narrative-driven: The meditation is typically led by a spoken narrative, which can be delivered in person by a meditation teacher or via audio recordings, apps, or videos.

Thematic Focus: Many guided meditations are centered around specific themes such as calmness, gratitude, or physical relaxation. They may also target specific outcomes like improving sleep, reducing anxiety, or enhancing self-esteem.

Sensory Engagement: The guide often uses descriptive language to engage the senses, helping the practitioner visualize scenarios, imagine sensations like warmth or light, or focus on the breath or body parts.

Indicative Process of Guided Meditation

Here's how you can engage in guided meditation:

1. Selecting a Guided Meditation: Choose a guided meditation that fits your needs. This could be based on length, the focus of the meditation, or the voice and style of the guide. There are numerous resources available online, including meditation apps, YouTube channels, podcasts, and local wellness centers.
2. Creating a Conducive Environment: To get the most out of guided meditation, find a quiet and comfortable space where you can relax without interruptions. You can sit or lie down, depending on your comfort and the nature of the meditation.
3. Using Audio or Video Tools: Play the guided meditation using whatever device is most convenient for you. This could be through headphones on your smartphone, a computer, or

a speaker system, depending on your preference for privacy or immersion.

4. Following the Guidance: Close your eyes and listen as the guide leads you through the session. Follow the instructions as closely as possible. This might involve visualizing images, focusing on your breath, or mentally scanning different parts of your body.
5. Engaging Actively: While the guide provides direction, it's important for you to engage actively with the process. This means mentally participating in the visualizations and thinking actively about the sensations, emotions, and thoughts that the guide suggests.
6. Reflecting Post-Meditation: After the guided session ends, take a few moments to reflect on the experience. Think about how you feel now compared to before the meditation. This can help deepen your practice and make mental notes of what works best for you.

Guided meditation can be a powerful tool for mental relaxation and emotional regulation. It's especially beneficial for individuals who find it challenging to silence their mind independently or who enjoy a more structured approach to meditation.

Vipassana Meditation

Vipassana, which means "to see things as they really are," is one of India's most ancient techniques of meditation. It was taught in India more than 2500 years ago as a universal remedy for universal ills. The practice was reintroduced by S.N. Goenka in the 20th century and has spread globally. The practice aims at purifying the mind by eliminating the causes of suffering: craving, aversion, and ignorance. Practitioners learn to observe the interplay of body sensations and mind, with a balanced awareness and understanding of impermanence, which leads to a profound experiential wisdom of the true nature of reality.

Vipassana meditation is a powerful practice for developing mindfulness and gaining deep insights into the nature of reality. By consistently observing your breath and bodily sensations and noting the arising and passing of thoughts and emotions, you can cultivate a greater sense of peace, clarity, and understanding.

Process of Vipassana Meditation

Vipassana Meditation, also known as Insight Meditation, is a traditional Buddhist practice aimed at cultivating mindfulness and insight into the true nature of reality. This is an indicative process.

1. Find a Quiet Space: Choose a calm and quiet place where you can sit undisturbed. This helps minimize distractions and enhances concentration.
2. Assume a Comfortable Posture: Sit in a comfortable position. You can sit cross-legged on a cushion, in a chair with your feet flat on the ground, or in any position where you can stay still and relaxed for an extended period. Keep your back straight but not rigid, hands resting comfortably on your lap or knees.
3. Close Your Eyes and Relax: Close your eyes to help focus inward. Take a few deep breaths to relax your body and mind, settling into your posture.
4. Focus on Your Breath: Direct your attention to the natural rhythm of your breath. Observe the sensation of the breath as it enters and leaves your nostrils, or the rising and falling of your abdomen. Do not try to control your breathing; simply observe it as it is.
5. Maintain Mindful Awareness: As you focus on your breath, you may notice your mind starting to

wander. This is normal. When you become aware that your mind has wandered, gently bring your attention back to the breath. The key is to observe without judgment. Acknowledge the thoughts, feelings, or sensations that arise and then return to the breath.

6. Expand Your Awareness: Gradually, expand your focus from your breath to include other bodily sensations, sounds, and thoughts. Observe these sensations and thoughts with the same mindful awareness, noting them without attachment or aversion. You can use mental notes such as "thinking," "hearing," "itching," etc., to identify and acknowledge these experiences.
7. Deepen Your Insight: As you practice, try to observe the impermanent nature of all experiences. Notice how sensations, thoughts, and emotions arise and pass away. This helps cultivate insight into the nature of impermanence, suffering, and non-self. Be aware of the present moment and accept it as it is, without clinging or resistance.
8. Conclude the Session: After your meditation session (which can last anywhere from 10 to 60 minutes), gradually bring your attention back to your body and surroundings. Open your eyes slowly and take a few moments to sit quietly, reflecting on your practice and any insights gained.

Vipassana Meditation Effectiveness

- Consistency: Regular practice is essential for developing mindfulness and insight. Aim to meditate daily, even if only for a short period.
- Patience: Vipassana is a gradual practice. Be patient with yourself and the process, allowing insights to develop naturally over time.
- Mindful Living: Try to carry the mindfulness cultivated during meditation into your daily activities, maintaining awareness and presence in everything you do.

For more structured guidance, consider attending a Vipassana meditation retreat or course, where experienced teachers can provide detailed instructions and support. Online resources and books by experienced practitioners can also be valuable aids in deepening your practice.

Vipassana Meditation Course

Vipassana is typically taught through a structured 10-day residential course, which includes the following steps:

- Code of Discipline: Participants agree to follow a strict code of discipline, which includes abstaining from all forms of communication with fellow participants, not using any electronic devices, and abstaining from any form of entertainment or distraction.

- Noble Silence: Silence is observed for the majority of the course, which means no verbal communication, gestures, or eye contact, to help focus inwardly and work diligently on one's meditation.
- Anapana Meditation: The first few days are focused on Anapana meditation, which involves focusing attention on the breath as it enters and exits the nostrils. This serves to sharpen the mind in preparation for the practice of Vipassana.
- Vipassana Meditation: Around the fourth day, the practice of Vipassana begins. Practitioners start observing sensations throughout the body, understanding their impermanent nature without reacting to them. The technique teaches "equanimity", calm mental reactions to experiences, regardless of whether they are pleasant or unpleasant.
- Metta Bhavana: The final day of the retreat focuses on Metta Bhavana, or loving-kindness meditation, which involves cultivating feelings of goodwill and kindness towards all beings. This practice helps to balance the mind after intense days of self-observation.

- Daily Discourses: Each evening, a discourse is given by Shri Goenka (via video recordings), which explains the process, provides encouragement, and offers theoretical context to what the students are practicing.
- Interviews with Teacher: Throughout the course, opportunities are provided to ask questions and receive personal guidance from the teacher, to clarify any doubts and ensure the technique is practiced correctly.
- Integration: Post-retreat, practitioners are encouraged to continue the practice daily to maintain and deepen the benefits of Vipassana. Regular practice helps integrate the insights and mental discipline into everyday life.

Practicing Vipassana meditation is challenging but often described as life-transforming, as it profoundly changes one's understanding of oneself and one’s reactions to the world. It is advised to learn Vipassana from a qualified teacher at a dedicated retreat to fully understand and correctly practice the technique under guided supervision.

Zen Meditation (Zazen)

Zen meditation, or Zazen, is a form of meditation that is a central practice in Zen Buddhism. The term "Zazen" literally means "seated meditation" and emphasizes quieting the mind and body to experience insight into the nature of existence and to cultivate an awareness of one's true self. It is practiced in Zen temples and monasteries worldwide and is a pathway to achieving inner peace and enlightenment.

Characteristics of Zen Meditation

- Posture: The physical posture is considered crucial in Zazen. Practitioners typically sit in the lotus or half-lotus position, though other positions are also acceptable as long as the back is straight and the mind alert.
- Breathing: Special attention is given to breathing deeply from the hara (the center of gravity in the lower abdomen) and maintaining a focus on rhythmic breathing.

- Mindfulness: Practitioners are encouraged to let go of all distracting thoughts and sensations, focusing on the present moment and maintaining an awareness of the environment and one's thoughts without attachment.

Indicative Process of Zen Meditation (Zazen)

1. Finding a Space: Choose a quiet and uncluttered space. Traditionally, Zazen is practiced in a clean room facing a wall to minimize external distractions.
2. Sitting Posture: Sit on a cushion or chair. If using a cushion, sit on the forward third of it. The most common postures include the full lotus, half-lotus, Burmese (simple cross-legged), or seiza (kneeling). The key is to keep the back straight, with the spine in its natural position.
3. Hand Position: Place your hands in the cosmic mudra. This involves placing your dominant hand palm up on your lap, then placing the other hand palm up on top of the dominant hand, and finally touching the tips of the thumbs together to form an oval frame.
4. Eyes: Keep your eyes open or half-open. Gazing downward about a meter in front of you helps reduce daydreaming or drowsiness, which are common in meditation.

5. Breathing: Focus on your breathing, which should be natural and relaxed, yet deep and quiet. The emphasis is often on exhaling deeply and then letting the inhalation occur naturally.
6. Clearing the Mind: Try to clear your mind of all thoughts and ideas. When thoughts arise, acknowledge them without attachment and gently return your focus to your breath or a "koan" if used (a paradoxical anecdote or riddle used in Zen practice to provoke deeper thinking).
7. Duration: Beginners might start with 5-10 minutes of Zazen and gradually increase the time as they get more comfortable. Experienced practitioners may sit for periods of 30 minutes to an hour at a time.
8. Ending the Session: Gently sway your body from side to side in increasing arcs before slowly stretching out your legs. This helps in bringing the body out of the meditation posture gradually.

Zazen is less about achieving specific insights or experiences and more about settling into the process and cultivating a state of open, alert awareness. The practice is often described as a way to learn how to sit with what is, without expectation or attachment. Regular practice is said to cultivate deep inner calm, emotional stability, and increased insight into the nature of existence.

Progressive Relaxation

Progressive relaxation, also known as progressive muscle relaxation (PMR), is a technique that involves systematically tensing and then relaxing different muscle groups in the body. It is based on the principle that physical relaxation can lead to mental relaxation, which is beneficial in reducing stress, anxiety, and improving overall well-being. This technique was developed by Dr. Edmund Jacobson in the early 1920s, who theorized that since muscle tension accompanies anxiety, one can reduce anxiety by learning how to relax the muscular tension.

In the context of meditation, progressive relaxation serves as a preparatory practice that helps to calm the mind and ease the body into a state of deep relaxation and heightened awareness. It is often used at the beginning of a meditation session to help facilitate a smoother transition into deeper meditative states.

Indicative Process of Progressive Relaxation

1. Find a Quiet Environment: Choose a quiet, comfortable space where you will not be disturbed. This can be any place where you can sit or lie down comfortably without external distractions.
2. Comfortable Position: Sit or lie down in a comfortable position. You can use a mat, a bed, or any soft surface. If sitting, ensure your back is supported and upright. If lying down, lay flat on your back with your legs uncrossed and arms relaxed at your sides.
3. Start with Deep Breathing: Begin by taking several deep breaths. Inhale slowly through your nose, allowing your chest and lower belly to rise, and then exhale slowly through your mouth. Deep breathing helps initiate the relaxation process.
4. Tense and Relax Muscle Groups: Start at your feet and work your way up to your face, or vice versa. Tense each muscle group vigorously, but not to the point of strain, and maintain this tension for about 5 seconds. Then, abruptly release the tension in that muscle group. Focus on the changes you feel when the tension is released. Spend about 10 to 20 seconds relaxing, and then move on to the next muscle group.
5. Muscle Groups Sequence:
   - Feet: Curl your toes downward to create tension in your foot. Hold and release.

- Legs: Tighten your calf muscles by pulling toes towards you. Hold and release. Then, do the same with your thigh muscles.
- Hands: Clench your fists. Hold and release.
- Arms: Tense your biceps by drawing your forearms up towards your shoulders and “making a muscle” with both arms. Hold and release.
- Buttocks: Tighten by pulling your buttocks together. Hold and release.
- Stomach: Tighten your stomach muscles by sucking your stomach in. Hold and release.
- Chest: Take a deep breath and hold it, tightening the muscles. Hold and release.
- Neck and Shoulders: Raise your shoulders up to touch your ears (shrug). Hold and release.
- Face: Make a frowning face, scrunching your eyes and lips. Hold and release.

6. Return to Deep Breathing: Once you have moved through all the muscle groups, return to deep breathing. Feel the sensation of calmness and relaxation spread through your body.
7. Mindfulness or Silent Meditation: Transition into a state of mindfulness or another form of silent meditation. The deep physical relaxation achieved can help facilitate a deeper mental state of meditation.

8. Conclude with Awareness: Gently bring your awareness back to the room. Wiggle your fingers and toes, stretch if needed, and open your eyes. Take a moment to notice how your body feels.

Progressive relaxation can greatly enhance the quality of meditation by reducing physical tension that can often hinder mental relaxation. This technique is especially useful for those new to meditation or those who find it difficult to sit still and quiet the mind due to physical discomforts.

Body Scan Meditation

Body scan meditation is a form of mindfulness meditation where you mentally scan your body from head to toe, observing and noticing areas of tension, pain, warmth, or relaxation without trying to change anything. This practice helps to cultivate moment-to-moment awareness of the body and serves as a simple method to reconnect with the physical self and release physical and emotional tension. It is often used as a way to help the mind quiet and to recover from stress, anxiety, and pain.

Characteristics of Body Scan Meditation

- Mindfulness-based: The body scan is grounded in mindfulness principles, focusing on physical sensations and experiences.
- Systematic: The meditation involves a sequential process, typically starting at one end of the body (often the feet) and methodically moving to the other (the head), paying attention to various parts of the body.

- Non-judgmental Observation: It emphasizes observing bodily sensations without judgment or the need to change anything. This practice helps to develop a deeper awareness of bodily sensations and a non-reactive relationship with one's physical experiences.

Indicative Process of Body Scan Meditation

Preparation: Find a quiet place where you can relax without interruptions. This meditation can be done lying down, sitting, or in other comfortable postures. Wear comfortable clothing and ensure a conducive environment for relaxation.

Starting Position: Lie on your back with your legs extended, a small pillow under your head, and your arms at your sides with palms facing up. If sitting, ensure your back is straight and your feet are flat on the floor.

Focus on Breathing: Take a few deep breaths to relax your body and mind. Notice the rhythm of your breath and allow it to become natural and steady.

Begin the Body Scan: Start at the toes of your feet. Focus your attention on any sensations you feel in that part of the body. It could be warmth, coolness, tingling, pressure, or nothing at all. Slowly move your attention from one part of the body to another, your feet, ankles, calves, knees, thighs, and so forth. Spend a few moments on each part.

Observation: As you focus on each part, acknowledge any sensations, pain, or discomfort. Notice how each part feels but without trying to change anything. The goal is not to relieve pain but to become aware of each moment and each part of your body.

Breathing into Sensations: If you encounter areas of tension or discomfort, imagine breathing into them, and then breathe out the tension. This can help in releasing the discomfort, though the primary aim remains awareness and acceptance.

Continue Scanning: Gradually move up through your body, from your feet to the top of your head. Pay attention to your lower back, abdomen, chest, hands, arms, shoulders, neck, face, and finally the top of your head.

Finishing the Meditation: Once you reach the top of your head, spend a few moments reviewing your body as a whole and observe the general feeling of calm and relaxation. Gently wiggle your fingers and toes to bring movement back into your body, stretch if necessary, and open your eyes when ready.

Body scan meditation can be particularly useful for identifying areas of chronic pain or tension and cultivating a deeper sense of bodily awareness. It is often used in mindfulness-based stress reduction programs to help decrease stress and improve emotional reactions to physical sensations.

Visualization Meditation

Visualization meditation, also known as guided imagery or creative visualization, is a meditation technique that involves intentionally imagining positive, meaningful, or peaceful scenes, situations, or results. This form of meditation leverages the power of the mind to influence emotions and physical states, promoting relaxation, stress reduction, and healing. It is often used to enhance a sense of peace, improve personal skills, overcome psychological hurdles, and visualize successful outcomes in various aspects of life.

Characteristics of Visualization Meditation

- Mental Imagery: The core element is the creation of vivid and detailed images in the mind. Practitioners are encouraged to use all their senses to make these visualizations as real as possible.
- Goal-Oriented: Often, visualization is used with specific goals in mind, such as improving performance in a sport, enhancing public

speaking skills, or achieving a state of calm in stressful situations.

- Emotional Engagement: By imagining positive outcomes or beautiful scenes, practitioners can elicit real emotional responses that have a profound effect on their mood and outlook.

Indicative Process of Visualization Meditation

1. Prepare the Environment: Choose a quiet place where you can relax without interruptions. Comfort is key as it helps in maintaining focus during visualization.
2. Comfortable Position: Sit or lie down in a comfortable position. You can sit in a meditation chair or cushion or lie on your back. Ensure your body is relaxed.
3. Relaxation: Begin with a few minutes of deep breathing to relax your mind and body. Breathe slowly and deeply, focusing on letting go of tension with each exhale.
4. Set an Intention: starting the visualization, set a clear intention or goal for your meditation. Decide what scene, outcome, or feeling you wish to visualize.
5. Begin Visualization: Close your eyes and start forming a mental image of your intention. Imagine

the scene as vividly as possible. Engage all your senses, sight, sound, smell, touch, and taste. For example, if you are visualizing a beach, see the sun setting over the ocean, hear the waves crashing, smell the salt water, feel the sand under your feet, and taste the salt in the air. Make the visualization as detailed and vivid as possible. The more real it feels, the more effective the meditation will be.

6. Maintain Focus: Keep your mind focused on the visualization. If your mind wanders, gently bring it back to the image and the sensations you are imagining.
7. Emotional Connection: Try to connect emotionally with the scene. Feel the joy, peace, or confidence that comes with the imagery. Allow these feelings to wash over you and take root in your mind and body.
8. Gradually Conclude: After spending a sufficient amount of time in your visualized scenario (usually 10-20 minutes, depending on your preference), slowly bring your mind back to your present surroundings. Take a few deep breaths, wiggle your fingers and toes, and when you're ready, open your eyes.
9. Reflect: Spend a few moments reflecting on the experience. Consider how you feel now compared to before the meditation. Think about

any insights or feelings that arose during the process.

Visualization meditation can be a powerful tool for personal development and emotional healing. By regularly practicing this form of meditation, you can enhance your mental clarity, improve your ability to focus, and foster a positive mindset that supports your overall well-being and success.

Gazing Meditation
(*Trataka*)

Trataka, or gazing meditation, is a form of concentration practice in traditional yoga, where the gaze is fixed on a single point or object to help focus the mind and develop concentration. This practice is known to purify the eyesight, strengthen the eye muscles, and improve mental clarity and concentration. Trataka can be performed on a variety of objects, but common choices include a candle flame, a black dot on the wall, or a small object like a crystal.

Characteristics of Trataka

- Single-Point Focus: The essence of Trataka is to maintain steady focus on a single visual point without blinking, until tears are produced.
- Stages of Practice: Initially performed with open eyes until they water, followed by closing the eyes and visualizing the object in the mind's eye, continuing to hold the focus.

- Cleansing Effect: It is considered a cleansing practice, or Kriya, in yoga that cleanses the eyes and stimulates the third eye or the ajna chakra, enhancing the practitioner's intuitive abilities.

Indicative Process of Gazing Meditation (Trataka)

1. Preparation: Choose a quiet, dimly lit room where you won't be disturbed. The dim lighting helps in focusing on the object without strain. Prepare your chosen object of focus. If using a candle, place it on a stable surface at eye level about an arm's length away.
2. Comfortable Seating: Sit in a comfortable meditation posture such as Padmasana (Lotus Position), Sukhasana (Easy Pose), or simply on a chair if floor sitting is uncomfortable. Ensure your spine is straight, and your body is relaxed.
3. Object Focus: Light the candle and gently fix your gaze on the flame. The flame should be steady and quiet without flickering. If using another object, ensure it is distinctly visible and steady. Try to keep your eyes open without blinking for as long as comfortable. The aim is to build your concentration and mental discipline.
4. Visualize After Closing Eyes: When you feel the need to blink, or your eyes begin to water, close your eyes gently. With your eyes closed, try to visualize the flame or object in your "mind's eye"

at the point between your eyebrows (the location of the third eye chakra). Maintain the image as clearly as possible.

5. Deepening the Practice: Focus on the after-image of the object as long as you can hold it in your vision. As it fades, bring it back with your eyes closed, continually strengthening your mental visualization. Once the image can no longer be held, gently open your eyes and repeat the process. This cycle can be repeated two to three times during a practice session.
6. Conclude the Session: by completing the cycles. Sit quietly for a few minutes in meditation, observing the effects of the practice on your mental state. You may notice enhanced mental clarity and a sense of calm.
7. Regular Practice: Regular practice of Trataka is recommended to reap full benefits, such as improved concentration and opening of the third eye. Over time, practitioners often experience profound improvements in both mental focus and inner perceptual abilities.

Trataka is a simple yet powerful practice that is accessible to people of all ages and can be a rewarding addition to a regular meditation routine, helping to enhance mental clarity and focus.

Sound Meditation

Sound meditation, also known as sound healing or sound bath meditation, is a meditative practice that involves using musical instruments or vocal sounds to create an immersive, resonant environment that promotes relaxation and healing. This practice leverages the therapeutic properties of sound vibrations to enhance mental clarity, emotional release, and physical relaxation.

The sounds used in this form of meditation can vary but typically include singing bowls (Tibetan or crystal), gongs, tuning forks, bells, and even human voices chanting or singing. The theory behind sound meditation is based on the idea that all matter (including the human body) is vibrating at specific frequencies, and these frequencies can be influenced positively by resonant external sounds.

Characteristics of Sound Meditation

- Vibrational Healing: The core mechanism at work in sound meditation is vibrational energy, which can influence the body's vibration and promote wellness.

- Passive Engagement: Unlike some forms of meditation that require active participation in visualizing or controlling the breath, sound meditation generally involves passively listening and absorbing the sound waves.
- Accessibility: It is highly accessible and easy to participate in, as it requires no prior meditation experience and can be particularly effective for those who find silent meditation challenging.

Indicative Process of Sound Meditation

1. Setting the Space: Choose a quiet and comfortable space where you will not be disturbed. This can be a dedicated meditation room or any quiet corner in your home or outdoors. Prepare the space by ensuring it is clean and possibly dimly lit to enhance relaxation. Some practitioners use aromatherapy or soft lighting to create a more immersive atmosphere.
2. Choosing Your Sound Medium: Decide on the sound instruments or recordings you will use. Tibetan singing bowls, crystal bowls, gongs, or prerecorded soundtracks are popular choices. If

attending a live sound meditation session, the facilitator will prepare the instruments.

3. Comfortable Position: Lie down or sit in a comfortable position. Using a yoga mat, cushions, or blankets can enhance your comfort, as you might be in the same position for an extended period (typically 20-60 minutes).
4. Beginning the Meditation: The facilitator or recording will begin playing the instruments. The sounds should start gently and gradually fill the space. Close your eyes and take a few deep breaths to relax your body. Allow yourself to feel grounded and present in the moment.
5. Engaging with the Sounds: Focus on the sounds you hear. Notice the quality, texture, and layers of the sounds without trying to analyze them. Allow the vibrations to wash over you, noticing any physical sensations or emotions that arise. Some people experience waves of emotion or physical sensations like tingling due to the vibrational impact of the sounds.
6. Deepening the Experience: As the meditation progresses, allow yourself to drift deeper into relaxation. It's normal for the mind to wander, but whenever you notice this, gently bring your attention back to the sounds.
7. Closing the Session: The session will typically wind down with a gradual reduction in the intensity and volume of the sounds, allowing you

to slowly come back to a state of normal awareness. Take your time to move or sit up. It's common to feel deeply relaxed or even slightly disoriented immediately after a sound bath.

8. Reflection and Integration: After the session, spend a few minutes in silence, reflecting on the experience. Many practitioners find it helpful to journal about their feelings and any insights that arose during the meditation.

Sound meditation can be a profound and transformative experience, offering benefits like reduced stress, enhanced sleep, and a deeper sense of peace and well-being. It's a unique form of meditation that appeals to those who appreciate sensory experiences and are open to exploring the healing power of sound.

Nature Meditation

Nature meditation involves meditating in the natural environment to harness the calming, rejuvenating qualities of nature, enhancing the meditation experience. This practice is based on the principle that being in nature can lower stress, improve mood, and enhance cognitive function. Nature meditation can take many forms, including walking in a forest, sitting by a stream, or simply being in a garden. It leverages the sights, sounds, and smells of the outdoors to facilitate deep relaxation and mindfulness.

Characteristics of Nature Meditation

- Sensory Engagement: Utilizes the natural environment to engage all senses, fostering a deep connection with the external world.
- Accessibility: Can be practiced in any natural setting, from a backyard to a mountain top, depending on what's available and convenient.
- Versatility: Includes various forms, such as mindful walking, sitting quietly in nature, or even

actively engaging in an activity like gardening with mindful awareness.

Indicative Process of Nature Meditation

1. <u>Choose Your Environment</u>: Select a natural setting that you find calming and accessible. This could be a park, a beach, a forest trail, or even your garden. Ensure the place is safe and conducive to relaxation and reflection.
2. <u>Prepare for the Session</u>: Dress appropriately for the environment and weather to stay comfortable. Bring any items you might need, such as water, a mat, or a portable chair, and perhaps insect repellent if you're in a bug-prone area.
3. <u>Settling In</u>: Once you arrive at your chosen spot, take a few moments to settle in. You can start by walking around gently to acclimate to the space. Find a spot where you feel comfortable to sit or stand. If you prefer, you can continue walking slowly throughout your session.
4. <u>Engage Your Senses</u>: Begin by closing your eyes and taking several deep breaths to transition into a state of mindfulness. Open your eyes and actively engage your senses. Notice the sights, the sounds, and the smells around you. Feel the air on your skin and the ground beneath you.

5. Mindfulness Practice: Focus on the present moment and your sensory experiences. If your mind wanders, gently bring your attention back to the natural beauty around you. If sitting, you might choose to focus on the rhythm of your breath or the sensations of the air moving around you. If walking, concentrate on the sensation of your feet touching the ground, the rhythm of your stride, and the feeling of movement.
6. Deepening the Meditation: Allow yourself to become fully immersed in the experience. You might find particular natural elements, like the sound of water or the wind in the trees, that particularly draw your attention. Focus deeply on these elements. Use the rhythm of nature, such as the waves against the shore or the wind rustling through leaves, to deepen your relaxation and mindfulness.
7. Concluding the Session: Gradually bring your meditation to a close. Take a few more deep breaths and perhaps express gratitude for the time spent in nature and the relaxation experienced. Slowly stand (if seated) and stretch your body, taking in the environment one last time before leaving.
8. Integration: As you leave, try to carry the calmness and mindfulness from your nature meditation into the rest of your day.

Nature meditation is a powerful way to connect with the environment and access the inherent soothing qualities of the natural world. This practice not only enhances personal well-being but also fosters a greater appreciation and respect for nature.

Color Meditation

Color meditation is a form of visualization meditation that focuses on different colors to influence mood, emotions, and even physiological responses. Each color is believed to carry specific energies and associations that can affect the mind and body in various ways. For instance, blue is often associated with calmness and serenity, while red might evoke feelings of energy and passion. This type of meditation leverages these color associations to achieve desired effects, such as relaxation, energization, or healing.

Characteristics of Color Meditation

- Use of Color as Focus: The primary focus in color meditation is a specific color visualized either in the mind's eye or by looking at objects of that color.
- Emotional and Psychological Impact: Different colors are thought to influence specific emotions and mental states, making this practice

particularly useful for addressing issues like stress, anxiety, or lack of focus.

- Enhances Visual Imagination: This practice can enhance one's ability to visualize and maintain concentration, strengthening the mind's eye and imaginative capabilities.

Indicative Process of Color Meditation

Preparation: Choose a quiet and comfortable space where you can sit or lie down without interruption. You may choose to dim the lights or use colored lights to enhance the sensory experience of the meditation.

Selecting a Color: Decide on a color that corresponds to the intention of your meditation. For example, select green for healing and balance, blue for calmness and peace, or yellow for energy and cheerfulness. You can have an object of that color in front of you, use a colored light, or simply visualize the color in your mind.

Settle Into a Comfortable Position: Sit comfortably with your back straight but relaxed. If lying down, ensure your body is symmetrically laid out for even energy distribution.

Begin with Deep Breathing: Start by taking deep, slow breaths to relax your body and clear your mind of distractions. This will prepare you for deeper concentration.

Visualization: Close your eyes and imagine the color you have chosen filling your vision. Visualize the color as a bright, dynamic energy engulfing your entire field of view. You can imagine the color as a mist or light surrounding you, filling the room, or emanating from your body.

Focus on the Color's Energy: Think about the qualities associated with the color. Feel its energy interacting with your body. Imagine it affecting your mood, emotions, and physical state in positive ways. Concentrate on how the color makes you feel. Notice any changes in your body, thoughts, or emotions as you focus on the color.

Deepen the Meditation: Continue to breathe deeply and allow yourself to be immersed in the color. If your mind wanders, gently bring your attention back to the color visualization.

Concluding the Session: Gradually bring your focus back to your regular state of awareness. Open your eyes when you feel ready, taking a moment to adjust to your surroundings. Reflect on the experience and any new sensations or feelings that arose during the meditation.

Integration: After completing the meditation, think about ways you can incorporate the color into your daily life to continue benefiting from its energies, such as wearing clothing of that color or using decor elements in your environment.

Color meditation is an accessible and versatile technique that can be tailored to individual needs and preferences, making it a valuable addition to one's meditative practices. It is particularly effective for those who are visually inclined and enjoy using imagery in their meditation routines.

Dance Meditation

Dance meditation, also known as movement meditation, combines the physicality of dance with the mindfulness of meditation. It is a form of active meditation where movement guides the meditation experience, allowing participants to express themselves freely through dance while focusing on their inner feelings and sensations. This practice helps in releasing physical tension, emotional stress, and enhances the connection between the mind and body.

Dance meditation is not about choreographed steps or technical skill, but rather about letting go of structured movement to allow natural, spontaneous expression. It is often used to explore and release emotions, enhance self-awareness, and achieve a state of mental clarity and peace.

Characteristics of Dance Meditation

- Freedom of Expression: Unlike traditional dance forms, dance meditation does not follow specific routines or steps. Participants move however they feel, allowing for a personal and introspective experience.

- Mind-Body Integration: It emphasizes the connection between physical movement and mental state, encouraging practitioners to explore how their bodies feel as they move and how movement influences their emotions and thoughts.
- Therapeutic Benefits: By combining dance and meditation, this practice offers both the mental benefits of meditation, such as reduced anxiety and increased focus, and the physical benefits of dance, including improved strength and flexibility.

Indicative Process of Dance Meditation

1. Setting the Space: Choose a safe and comfortable space where you can move freely without interruptions. This could be a room with enough space to dance around or a secluded outdoor area.
2. Prepare Yourself: Wear comfortable clothing that allows for unrestricted movement. You might choose to play music that you find calming or energizing, depending on your preference. Music can help facilitate movement and enhance the meditative experience.

3. Initial Relaxation: Begin with a few moments of stillness. Close your eyes, take deep breaths, and notice any areas of tension in your body. Use this time to transition from the external world into your internal experience.
4. Start to Move: Open your eyes and start moving slowly. Let your body guide you; there are no right or wrong movements in dance meditation. Focus on your breath and how different parts of your body feel as you move. Let your movements flow naturally with the rhythm of your breathing or the music.
5. Engage Deeply: Gradually allow your movements to become more expansive and expressive. Move in ways that feel good to you, exploring different speeds, rhythms, and patterns. Pay attention to any emotions or thoughts that arise as you dance. Acknowledge them and express them through your movements.
6. Mindfulness and Reflection: Throughout your dance, maintain an attitude of mindfulness. Observe your movements, the sensations in your body, and the emotions you are experiencing without judgment. If your mind wanders, gently bring your focus back to your movement and the physical sensations.
7. Winding Down: Gradually slow your movements and start to bring your session to a close. Move towards stillness, perhaps ending with some

gentle stretching or a few moments of seated meditation. Reflect on your experience. Consider what emotions and thoughts came up and how the session affected your mental and physical state.

8. Integration: Consider how you can carry the mindfulness and awareness cultivated during dance meditation into your everyday activities. This could influence how you manage stress, interact with others, or engage with your tasks.

Dance meditation is an effective way to explore the interconnectedness of mind and body, providing a dynamic way to practice meditation that can be particularly appealing to those who find stillness challenging or who thrive on physical expression.

Movement Meditation

Movement meditation, also known as dynamic meditation, integrates movement with the mental focus and spiritual experience typical of meditation. Unlike traditional meditation, which often involves stillness and seated postures, movement meditation uses fluid motions to engage the body fully, making it particularly beneficial for those who find peace and focus easier to achieve when in motion. This practice can encompass a variety of activities, including walking, dancing, Tai Chi, and even routine tasks performed mindfully.

The idea behind movement meditation is to cultivate mindfulness and presence through movement, grounding practitioners in their bodies and the present moment. This form of meditation can help reduce stress, increase physical strength and flexibility, improve mental focus, and foster a deeper connection with the self and the environment.

Characteristics of Movement Meditation

- Integration of Body and Mind: Movement meditation emphasizes a harmonious connection between the body and mind, enhancing both physical and mental awareness.

- Accessibility: It is accessible to people of all fitness levels and can be adapted to suit individual needs and preferences.
- Engagement with the Environment: Many forms of movement meditation encourage interaction with one's surroundings, making it a multisensory experience.

Indicative Process of Movement Meditation

1. Choose Your Form of Movement: Select a type of movement that you find calming and immersive. This could be anything from walking in nature, practicing yoga, performing Tai Chi, or even engaging in more structured dance movements. The key is to choose a movement that allows you to focus and maintain a meditative state while being physically active.
2. Prepare the Environment: If indoors, ensure the space is clear and safe for movement. If outdoors, choose a quiet, pleasant environment where you can move without distractions or interruptions. Consider the terrain and weather conditions if you choose an outdoor setting.

3. Begin with Intention: Start by setting an intention for your meditation. This could be anything from seeking calmness and clarity to cultivating gratitude or compassion. Take a few moments to breathe deeply and center yourself before you begin moving.
4. Engage in the Movement: Begin your chosen form of movement slowly, focusing on each motion and its impact on your body. Maintain awareness of your breath, syncing it with your movements whenever possible. This synchronization helps deepen the meditative quality of the practice.
5. Maintain Mindful Awareness: As you move, keep your attention focused on the present moment. Notice the sensations in your body, the rhythm of your breath, and your interaction with your surroundings. Whenever your mind wanders, gently bring your focus back to your movement and breathing.
6. Explore the Movement: Allow yourself to experiment with different speeds and patterns of movement. Notice how changes in your movement affect your mental and emotional state. Be open to experiencing the movement in whatever form it takes, without judgment or expectation.
7. Conclude with Reflection: Gradually slow your movements and come to a stop. Spend a few moments in stillness, reflecting on your

experience. Conclude your session with a few deep breaths, acknowledging your work and thanking yourself for the time spent in meditation.

8. Integration: Consider ways to integrate the mindfulness and calm achieved during your movement meditation into the rest of your day. Reflect on any insights or changes in perspective that may have arisen during your practice.

Movement meditation is a dynamic way to experience the benefits of meditation while also engaging the body physically, making it an excellent option for those who prefer a more active form of meditation or for those looking to add a mindful component to their physical activities.

Music Meditation

Music meditation involves using music as a tool to facilitate deeper meditation, focus the mind, and promote relaxation. The sound and vibrations from music can profoundly affect our emotional and psychological states, making music a powerful medium to enhance the meditation experience. This practice can involve listening to specific types of music that evoke peace and calmness, or it may involve more active participation like chanting or playing musical instruments.

The type of music used in meditation can vary widely, from classical compositions and nature sounds to specially composed meditation tracks and traditional chanting. The key is choosing music that resonates with the individual and aids in achieving a deeper state of relaxation and mindfulness.

Characteristics of Music Meditation

- Aural Focus: The practice centers around using auditory stimuli to maintain and deepen concentration.
- Emotional and Psychological Resonance: Music can bypass intellectual barriers and directly affect the subconscious, making it easier to achieve emotional and psychological responses conducive to deep meditation.
- Accessibility: Music meditation can be practiced almost anywhere and is easily accessible through various mediums, making it highly versatile and widely appealing.

Indicative Process of Music Meditation

1. Selection of Music: Choose music that you find soothing and free from distracting elements. This could be ambient music, classical tracks, nature sounds, or even slow, rhythmic instrumentals. The absence of lyrics is often recommended to avoid engaging the mind in active listening and interpretation.
2. Prepare the Environment: Find a quiet, comfortable place where you can relax without interruptions. Using headphones can enhance

the immersive experience and help block out external noise.

3. Comfortable Position: Sit or lie down in a comfortable position. Ensure your back is supported if sitting. The goal is to eliminate any physical distractions that might detract from your focus on the music.
4. Begin with Deep Breathing: Start with a few deep breaths to relax your body and calm your mind. This helps prepare you for a deeper meditation experience.
5. Engage with the Music: Play the music at a comfortable volume. Close your eyes and focus your attention on the sound. Listen to the nuances of the music—the instruments, the melody, the rhythms. Allow the music to fill your awareness, letting other thoughts and concerns fade away. If your mind wanders, gently bring your attention back to the music.
6. Deepen Your Meditation: As you become more absorbed in the music, let it guide your inner experience. You might visualize scenes that the music evokes, feel the vibrations in your body, or simply drift in the auditory landscape the music creates.
7. Conclude the Session: Gradually let the music fade away, bringing your session to a close. If using a playlist, choose a track that naturally tapers off into silence. Take a moment to sit in

silence and stillness, observing any new sensations or emotions that have arisen during your session.

8. Reflect and Ground Yourself: Before getting up, reflect on the experience. How do you feel now compared to before you started? What did you notice during the meditation? Slowly bring your awareness back to your surroundings. Stretch gently if needed and open your eyes when you're ready.

Music meditation can be a deeply relaxing and spiritually enriching practice, especially for those who connect naturally with music. It offers a unique path to achieving mindfulness and tranquility, making it a popular choice in the diverse spectrum of meditation practices.

Nada Yoga

Nada Yoga is an ancient Indian spiritual practice that views sound as a pathway to enlightenment. The term "Nada" translates to "sound" or "tone," and in the context of Nada Yoga, it refers specifically to the internal sounds or mystical sounds heard during deep meditation. This practice is based on the premise that the universe and all its contents are composed of vibrations. Nada Yoga seeks to tune into these vibrations through the focus on sound, ultimately leading to a connection with one's higher self or the universal spirit.

Nada Yoga incorporates elements of both music and meditation, using sound as the primary tool to calm the mind and elevate consciousness. It is believed that by tuning into the sounds of the universe (including silence), one can transcend the physical boundaries of the world and reach higher states of awareness.

Characteristics of Nada Yoga

- Internal Sound Concentration: Practitioners focus on the sounds produced within the body and mind as a form of meditation.
- Integration of Sound and Breath: Sound vibrations are often synchronized with breathing techniques to deepen the meditative state.
- Spiritual Connection Through Sound: The ultimate goal is to experience the inner mystical sound (Anahata Nada), which leads to spiritual awakening.

Indicative Process of Nada Yoga

1. Preparation and Environment: Choose a quiet, comfortable place where you are unlikely to be disturbed. This practice can be done sitting on the floor with a cushion or on a chair with your feet flat on the ground. Ensure you are in comfortable clothing and have set aside sufficient time to not feel rushed.
2. Begin with Deep Breathing: Start by taking a few deep breaths to relax your body and calm your mind. Focus on inhaling deeply through the nose and exhaling slowly through the mouth. As you settle into a rhythmic breathing pattern, start to

let go of external worries and focus solely on the present moment.

3. Ahata and Anahata Sounds: Begin by listening to external sounds (Ahata Nada), such as the sound of your breath, ambient noises in the room, or gentle music if preferred. This helps the mind to initially focus and become more receptive to finer sounds. Gradually shift your focus to internal sounds (Anahata Nada). These may include sounds heard in the absence of external stimuli, like ringing, buzzing, or humming sounds perceived within the ears or head. Reaching to this level may require certain level of practice.
4. Deepening the Practice: Continue to focus on any internal sounds, letting them draw you deeper into meditation. It is important not to force the sounds but to let them come naturally. As you focus more on these sounds, your mind should become calmer, and your awareness of external sounds will diminish.
5. Integration of Mantra Chanting: Some practitioners integrate mantra chanting into their Nada Yoga practice. Mantras can be chanted aloud at first, then whispered, and finally repeated silently. This progression helps to internalize the sound and focus the mind.
6. Conclude with Silence: After a period of focusing on internal sounds, allow yourself to sit in silence. Observe the effects of the meditation on your

mind and body. Reflect on any changes in your perception of sound or any new internal sounds that may have emerged during your practice.

7. Closing the Session: Gently bring your awareness back to your breathing and to the physical sensations of your body. Open your eyes slowly and give yourself a few minutes to adjust before getting up.

Practicing Nada Yoga can lead to profound peace and insight, making it a powerful tool for those seeking deep meditation and spiritual growth. It teaches practitioners to use sound as a means of quieting the mind and connecting with the subtle aspects of existence, promoting a profound inner peace and understanding.

Somatic Meditation

Somatic meditation focuses on the body's internal experience rather than external objects or breath as focal points. This form of meditation stems from the understanding that the body itself holds wisdom, memories, and intuitive knowledge that can guide personal growth and healing. It emphasizes bodily sensations and the cultivation of mindfulness centered on the physical experiences within the body.

The practice is based on the principle that by turning inward and deeply listening to the body, one can tap into a more profound, innate awareness that goes beyond the thinking mind. This approach is particularly beneficial for those seeking to heal from physical or emotional trauma, as it encourages a direct connection with sensations and feelings that are often overlooked or suppressed in traditional mindfulness practices.

Characteristics of Somatic Meditation

- Body-Centered: It utilizes the body's sensations as the primary focus of meditation, encouraging a deeper connection with the self.
- Introspective: This practice fosters an inward-looking perspective, enhancing self-awareness and self-regulation.
- Healing and Integrative: Somatic meditation is often used for therapeutic purposes, helping individuals integrate and heal emotional and physical traumas.

Indicative Process of Somatic Meditation

1. Find a Quiet Space: Choose a comfortable and quiet place where you can relax without interruptions. This setting should allow you to focus entirely on your internal experience.
2. Prepare Your Body: Sit or lie down in a comfortable position. Ensure that your posture supports relaxation but also keeps you sufficiently alert. Using cushions or blankets can help maintain comfort throughout the session.
3. Grounding: Begin by taking several deep breaths to center yourself. Focus on the weight of your body against the chair or floor and notice any

areas where your body contacts the surface beneath you.

4. Body Scan: Slowly direct your attention through different parts of your body. Start from your toes and move upwards, or vice versa. Notice any sensations, tensions, or discomfort without trying to change them. Pay particular attention to the nuances of sensations, whether they're textural (such as tingling, throbbing, or warmth), emotional (feelings that arise in different parts of the body), or energetic.
5. Deepen Your Awareness: As you notice sensations, allow yourself to feel them fully. If emotions arise, acknowledge and explore them with curiosity. This practice is about observing and experiencing without judgment or avoidance. Invite any areas of tightness or discomfort to relax, but rather than forcing relaxation, simply observe what happens when you bring awareness to these areas.
6. Integration: Continue to maintain a gentle, non-intrusive awareness of your body. Over time, this can help you develop a deeper intuitive connection with your body's needs and responses. As you become more accustomed to listening to your body, you may start to notice insights or intuitions that arise from within, providing guidance or clarity in your life.

7. Closing the Session: Conclude your meditation by taking a few deep, grounding breaths. Gently wiggle your fingers and toes to bring yourself back to the external world. Reflect on the experience, noting any discoveries or particular feelings that stood out during the session.
8. Regular Practice: Consistent practice is essential in deepening the connection with your somatic experience. Regular sessions can significantly enhance your ability to listen to and understand your body's subtle messages.

Somatic meditation is powerful for those who wish to develop a deeper, more harmonious relationship with their bodies. It fosters emotional healing and a profound sense of presence, making it a valuable practice for enhancing overall well-being and mindfulness.

Dynamic Meditation

Dynamic Meditation is a highly active and expressive form of meditation developed by the Indian mystic Osho. This meditation is designed to be intense and cathartic, aiming to free practitioners from ingrained emotional and psychological patterns. Dynamic Meditation involves a series of chaotic and rhythmic movements followed by periods of stillness and relaxation. The process encourages the expression of repressed feelings and emotions, thereby facilitating emotional release and personal transformation.

Characteristics of Dynamic Meditation

- Active and Expressive: Unlike traditional meditation practices that emphasize stillness and quiet, Dynamic Meditation involves vigorous movement and vocalization.
- Stages of Practice: The meditation is divided into five distinct stages, each designed to provoke and release different energies and emotions.

- Therapeutic Benefits: It is often used as a means to deal with deep-seated emotional issues, stress, and to foster personal growth and awareness.

Indicative Process of Dynamic Meditation

Dynamic Meditation is typically performed in the early morning when, as Osho suggested, "the whole of nature becomes alive, the night has gone, the sun is coming up and everything becomes conscious and alert."

Preparation: Find a quiet and spacious area where you can move freely without inhibition. This practice requires privacy and space due to its vigorous nature. Wear comfortable clothing that allows for unrestricted movement.

First Stage- Breathing (10 minutes): Begin by breathing chaotically through the nose, concentrating always on the exhalation. The body should follow the rhythm of your breathing, allowing it to move as needed. Continue until you literally become the breathing, allowing it to be wild and free.

Second Stage- Explosive Movement (10 minutes): Explode! Let go of everything that needs to be thrown out. Follow your body. Give it freedom to express whatever is there. Go totally mad—scream, shout, cry, jump, shake, dance, sing, laugh; throw yourself around.

Hold nothing back; keep your whole body moving. A little acting often helps to get started. Never allow your mind to interfere with what is happening.

Third Stage- Hopping (10 minutes): With arms raised above your head, jump up and down shouting the mantra, "Hoo! Hoo! Hoo!" as deeply as possible, landing on the flats of your feet. Let the sound penetrate deep into the sex center. Give all you have; exhaust yourself completely.

Fourth Stage- Freeze (15 minutes): STOP! Freeze wherever you are, in whatever position you find yourself. Don't arrange the body in any way. A cough, a movement, anything will dissipate the energy flow and the effort will be lost. Be a witness to everything that is happening to you.

Fifth Stage: Celebration (15 minutes): Celebrate and rejoice through dance, expressing your gratitude towards the whole. Carry your happiness and peace with you throughout the day.

Dynamic Meditation is a profound technique that involves physical stress and the sudden cessation of that stress, a powerful method for accessing deeper emotional layers and rejuvenating the entire psyche. Regular practice is said to result in increased energy, improved health, and greater peace of mind, along with profound insights into one's behavior and psychological patterns.

Gratitude Meditation

Gratitude meditation is a mindful practice focused on expressing gratitude for the things in one's life, both big and small. This type of meditation cultivates an attitude of appreciation and thankfulness, which has been linked to a variety of positive health outcomes, including increased happiness, reduced depression, and better sleep. The practice involves reflecting on the aspects of your life that you are grateful for, thereby shifting attention away from negative or stressful thoughts to positive affirmations.

Characteristics of Gratitude Meditation

- Positive Focus: Centers on positive emotions associated with being thankful for what one has, rather than focusing on lacks or wants.
- Psychological Benefits: Known to enhance mental health by increasing positivity, improving self-esteem, and reducing stress and anxiety.

- Simplicity: Easy to practice and can be integrated into daily routines without needing special equipment or a lot of time.

Indicative Process of Gratitude Meditation

1. Find a Quiet Space: Choose a calm and comfortable place where you won't be interrupted. This could be a specific room in your home, a peaceful outdoor spot, or any place where you can sit quietly for a few minutes.
2. Prepare to Meditate: Sit in a comfortable position. You can sit on a chair, cushion, or on the floor, ensuring your back is straight but relaxed. Close your eyes to block out external visual stimuli and help internal focus.
3. Start with Deep Breathing: Begin by taking several deep breaths to relax your body and mind. Inhale slowly through your nose, allowing your chest and belly to rise, and exhale gently, feeling a sense of relaxation spreading throughout your body.
4. Reflect on Gratitude: Shift your focus to thinking about things you are grateful for. Start with broad aspects such as your health, family, or friends. Move on to more specific events of the day or week, such as a good meal, a productive meeting, or a pleasant interaction with someone. For each

item you think of, pause and reflect on how it benefits your life and why you are thankful for it.

5. Deepen Your Reflection: As you contemplate each aspect of gratitude, try to truly feel the gratitude. Notice any sensations in your body, perhaps warmth, a smile, or a sense of expansiveness. If your mind wanders or negative thoughts intrude, gently acknowledge them and bring your focus back to gratitude.
6. Use of Affirmations: You can also incorporate gratitude affirmations into your meditation, repeating phrases like "I am thankful for the abundance in my life," or "I appreciate the simple joys around me."
7. Conclude with a Gratitude Commitment: Finish your meditation by setting an intention to carry this sense of gratitude throughout your day. Slowly bring your attention back to your surroundings and open your eyes when you're ready.
8. Regular Practice: Regularly practicing gratitude meditation can profoundly impact your outlook and interaction with the world. Consider making it a daily routine, possibly at the beginning or end of your day, to cultivate a lasting sense of thankfulness.

Gratitude meditation is a simple yet powerful practice that can shift your perspective, enhance your well-being, and deepen your connections with others. By regularly acknowledging and appreciating the good in your life, you can foster a more positive and fulfilling life experience.

Intuitive Meditation

Intuitive Meditation is a practice that focuses on cultivating and enhancing one's inner intuitive abilities through meditation. Unlike more structured forms of meditation that might focus on the breath, a mantra, or specific visualization techniques, intuitive meditation is more about creating a space to listen deeply to one's own inner guidance and wisdom. This type of meditation encourages a dialogue with the subconscious mind, often leading to insights, creative ideas, and deeper understanding of one's own needs and desires.

Characteristics of Intuitive Meditation

- Flexibility: There is no strict protocol or guidelines to follow, making it highly adaptable to individual needs and moments.
- Inner Focus: The practice centers on tuning into internal experiences, sensations, and the subtle intuitive pulls rather than external stimuli.
- Enhances Self-Knowledge: By focusing inward, practitioners often develop a deeper understanding of themselves and their personal truth.

Indicative Process of Intuitive Meditation

1. Setting the Space: Choose a quiet and comfortable place where you can relax without interruptions. This setting is crucial as external disturbances can distract from the inward focus necessary for intuitive meditation.
2. Relax and Ground: Sit or lie in a comfortable position. Close your eyes and take a few deep breaths to ground yourself and calm your mind. Feel the weight of your body supported by the ground beneath you, letting go of any tension.
3. Invite Intuition: As you settle into a relaxed state, mentally or verbally invite your intuition to come forward. You might use a phrase like, "I open myself to my inner wisdom," or simply set an intention to listen.
4. Listen Deeply: Continue to breathe deeply and maintain a passive awareness of any thoughts, feelings, or sensations that arise. The key here is not to force anything but rather to allow your subconscious mind to speak. You might receive insights in the form of images, words, emotions, or physical sensations. Note these without judgment and without trying to interpret them right away.
5. Maintain Openness: Stay open to the experience, even if you feel like nothing is happening. Sometimes, intuition is subtle, and insights can come after the meditation during the day.

6. Dialogue with Your Inner Self: If you feel moved, you can ask questions internally and see what responses come up. Treat it like a conversation where you are both asking and listening for the answers within.
7. Closing the Session: When you feel the session is complete, gently begin to bring your awareness back to your physical surroundings. Take a few deep breaths, wiggle your fingers and toes, and when ready, open your eyes.
8. Reflect and Record: After the meditation, spend some time reflecting on any insights or feelings that arose. It can be helpful to journal about your experience to help process and remember what came through.
9. Regular Practice: Regular practice enhances the connection to your intuition. Try to incorporate intuitive meditation into your daily or weekly routine to continue developing your inner listening skills.

Intuitive meditation is a powerful tool for those looking to deepen their understanding of themselves and enhance their decision-making and creative processes. It helps foster a profound connection with the inner self, making it easier to navigate life's challenges with insight and clarity.

Third Eye Meditation

Third Eye Meditation focuses on the "third eye" chakra, which is traditionally located on the forehead between the eyebrows. This spot is often associated with insight, intuition, and a gateway to higher consciousness. In various spiritual traditions, especially within Hinduism and Buddhism, the third eye is seen as a mystical inner eye which provides perception beyond ordinary sight.

Characteristics of Third Eye Meditation

- Enhanced Intuition and Insight: The practice is believed to awaken psychic abilities and deepen one's intuitive insights.
- Focus on the Forehead Center: Concentration is primarily on the third eye chakra, envisaged as the seat of wisdom and the bridge to spiritual realms.
- Visualization: Involves visualizing an indigo light or energy at the third eye to stimulate this energy center.

Indicative Process of Third Eye Meditation

- Preparation: Find a quiet, comfortable place where you can sit without disturbances. Good posture is crucial; sit in a traditional meditation pose or in a chair with your feet flat on the ground and your spine upright.
- Relaxation: Begin with a few minutes of deep breathing to relax your body and calm your mind. Inhale deeply and exhale slowly, letting go of any tension in your body.
- Concentration on the Third Eye: Gently focus your attention on the point between your eyebrows. Imagine a spinning wheel of indigo light or simply focus on the physical sensations that you observe in that area, such as lightness, tingling, or warmth.
- Visualization: Visualize a third eye in the center of your forehead. Imagine it slowly opening, revealing an inward eye that sees beyond physical reality. You can visualize this eye as emitting a beam of light that illuminates your path to higher consciousness. Keep your physical eyes closed and let your awareness dwell in the space between your eyebrows. The goal is not to strain your physical eyes but to relax into the visualization.

- Deepening the Meditation: Continue to breathe slowly and deeply, maintaining your focus on the third eye. If your mind wanders, gently bring your focus back to the indigo light or the sensation at your forehead. Allow yourself to be absorbed by the experience, receiving any images, insights, or feelings that arise.
- Ending the Session: Gradually withdraw your focus from the third eye and become aware of your regular breathing pattern. Notice the overall stillness of your body and the calmness of your mind. Slowly open your eyes and take a moment to adjust to your surroundings.
- Reflect: Spend a few moments reflecting on the experience. People often find insights or creative ideas emerging from third eye meditation sessions. Consider keeping a meditation journal to record your experiences and any visions or insights that arise.
- Regular Practice: Consistent practice can enhance the benefits of third eye meditation. It's recommended to meditate daily or several times a week to develop and strengthen your third eye chakra.

Third Eye Meditation is a profound tool for those seeking to enhance their spiritual connectivity and psychic health. It promotes not only a greater sense of internal balance but also opens up avenues to deeper understanding and intuition. Regular practice is key to gaining the most from third eye meditation, as it deepens and strengthens the connections with the subtle energies of the body.

Chakra Meditation

Chakra meditation is a form of meditation that focuses on seven main chakras (energy centers) in the body to enhance and balance their energy flow. Originating from ancient Indian philosophy, chakras are seen as vital points of energy that govern physical, emotional, and spiritual functions. Chakra meditation aims to clear these energy centers from any blockages to promote health, wellbeing, and a harmonious balance within the body and mind.

Characteristics of Chakra Meditation

- Holistic Health: Each chakra is associated with different aspects of health and consciousness. By meditating on these chakras, one aims to achieve a balanced body, mind, and spirit.
- Energy Focus: The practice involves focusing on the flow of energy in the body and visualizing this energy moving through the chakras.
- Visualization: This form of meditation often uses vivid visualizations of colors and light

corresponding to each chakra, enhancing focus and engagement during meditation.

Indicative Process of Chakra Meditation

1. Preparation: Find a quiet, comfortable space where you won't be disturbed. This helps in maintaining focus and deepening the meditation experience. Sit in a comfortable position with your spine straight. You can sit on a chair, a meditation cushion, or on the floor in a cross-legged position.
2. Grounding: Start by taking deep breaths to center and ground yourself. Inhale slowly and deeply through your nose, then exhale through your mouth. Continue for a few minutes until you feel calm and present.
3. Opening the Chakras:
    - Begin with the root chakra located at the base of your spine. Visualize a vibrant red color at this spot and focus on feelings of stability and security.
    - Gradually move your focus up to the sacral chakra just below the navel, visualized with an orange glow. Concentrate on creativity and emotional balance.

- Proceed to the solar plexus chakra, visualizing a bright yellow color and focusing on feelings of confidence and control.
- Move up to the heart chakra, imagining a green light and focusing on love and compassion.
- Focus on the throat chakra next, visualizing a blue light, and think about communication and self-expression.
- Move your focus to the third eye chakra, between your eyebrows, visualizing an indigo light, concentrating on intuition and clarity of thought.
- Finally, focus on the crown chakra at the top of your head, visualizing a violet light, representing spiritual connection and enlightenment.

4. Balancing Energy: Visualize energy flowing effortlessly from the root chakra up through each chakra along the spine to the crown chakra. Imagine this energy as a bright white light, purifying and energizing every chakra. Spend several minutes visualizing this energy movement, ensuring that each chakra is engaged and cleared of any blockages.
5. Concluding the Meditation:

    - After spending time on each chakra, allow your focus to slowly return to your entire body.
    - Notice any sensations or emotions and acknowledge them without judgment.
    - Take a few deep breaths, and when you feel ready, gently open your eyes.
6. Reflection: Take some time to reflect on your experience. You might find it helpful to journal about what sensations, thoughts, or emotions arose during the meditation.
7. Regular Practice: Regular chakra meditation can help maintain the balance and flow of energy in your body. Consider incorporating it into your daily or weekly routine to maximize its benefits.

Chakra meditation is a deeply enriching practice that can enhance physical, emotional, and spiritual wellbeing. By focusing on and balancing the chakras, practitioners can foster greater harmony and peace in their lives.

Yoga Meditation

Yoga meditation is a form of meditation deeply rooted in the yogic tradition, which integrates the physical postures (asanas) of yoga with mindfulness and focused concentration. This practice is designed to harmonize the body and mind, enhancing overall well-being through a series of steps that guide the practitioner into a deep state of relaxation and heightened awareness. The ultimate goal of yoga meditation is not just physical improvement but also reaching a higher state of consciousness and self-realization.

Characteristics of Yoga Meditation

- Integrative Practice: Combines physical postures, controlled breathing, and meditation or relaxation.
- Mind-Body Connection: Emphasizes awareness and control of breath to enhance the connection between the mind and body.
- Spiritual Development: Often includes components of spiritual growth, such as

chanting, mantra repetition, and focusing on chakras (energy centers in the body).

Indicative Process of Yoga Meditation

1. Preparation: Find a quiet, comfortable space where you can practice without interruptions. Ensure the area is large enough to accommodate physical movement. Wear comfortable clothing that allows flexibility and free movement.
2. Begin with Physical Postures: Start with gentle yoga postures to prepare your body for seated meditation. This might include poses such as Cat-Cow for spinal flexibility, Forward Bend for stretching the back, or Child's Pose for relaxation. Focus on your breathing as you move into and hold each pose, aiming for smooth, even breaths.
3. Transition to Seated Postures: After completing the physical postures, transition to a seated position that is comfortable for a prolonged period. Common positions include Lotus Pose, Half-Lotus, or a simple cross-legged position. Ensure your back is straight, which helps in maintaining alertness during meditation.
4. Pranayama (Breathing Exercises): Engage in pranayama, or controlled breathing techniques, to stabilize your mind and bring your focus

inward. Techniques like Ujjayi Breath (Ocean Breath) or Anulom Vilom (Alternate Nostril Breathing) are popular for their calming effects.

5. Concentration and Meditation: Begin to narrow your focus to a single point of concentration. This could be the breath, a mantra, a visual object, or the sensation of energy at one of the chakras. As you focus, try to let go of other thoughts, bringing your mind back to the point of focus whenever it wanders.
6. Deep Meditation: Continue to deepen your meditation, staying in this phase for as long as you feel comfortable, ideally for at least 15-20 minutes. During this time, you may enter a state of deep peace and relaxation where the mind becomes less active. Maintain an attitude of passive observation, witnessing your thoughts and sensations without attachment.
7. Closing the Session: Gradually bring your awareness back to the present moment. Begin by deepening your breath, slowly moving your fingers and toes, and gently opening your eyes. Stretch if needed and transition slowly out of your seated position.
8. Integration: Spend a few moments in quiet reflection on your experience. Consider jotting down any insights or feelings that arose during your meditation. Set an intention to carry the

calmness and mindfulness from your meditation into the rest of your day.

Yoga meditation is a comprehensive approach to mental and physical health, drawing on ancient practices to promote healing, balance, and tranquility in daily life. Regular practice helps develop discipline, enhances focus, and contributes to spiritual growth.

Laughing Meditation

Laughing meditation, often associated with Laughter Yoga, combines unconditional laughter with yogic breathing (Pranayama). The idea is that voluntary laughter provides the same physiological and psychological benefits as spontaneous laughter. The practice is based on the premise that the body cannot differentiate between fake and genuine laughter; both produce similar beneficial effects. Laughing meditation is used to release stress, enhance mood, increase oxygen intake, and encourage a state of joyful relaxation.

Characteristics of Laughing Meditation

- Stress Reduction: Laughter reduces levels of stress hormones and triggers the release of endorphins, promoting an overall sense of well-being.
- Community and Connection: Often practiced in groups, laughing meditation helps build a sense of connection and community among participants.

- Accessibility: Easy to perform and does not require any special equipment or physical ability, making it accessible to a wide range of people.

Indicative Process of Laughing Meditation

1. Warm-up: Begin with gentle warm-up exercises to loosen the muscles and prepare your body. This might include stretching, chanting, clapping, or rhythmic movements.
2. Breathing Exercises: Incorporate deep breathing exercises to relax the mind and body and prepare for laughter. This involves inhaling deeply through the nose and exhaling slowly through the mouth, often with a focus on the diaphragm.
3. Laughter Exercises: Start with intentional laughter, even if it feels forced at first, voluntary chuckles can turn into real laughter. This can be initiated through various activities, such as greeting each other with a laugh, telling a funny story, or even by making eye contact and playfully mimicking each other. Engage in exercises that promote childlike playfulness, which can help to stimulate natural laughter. Props like humorous hats or toys can be used to enhance the mood.
4. Cultivation of Playful Attitude: Maintain a playful, light-hearted attitude throughout the session.

This mindset helps reduce inhibitions and encourages a freer expression of joy.

5. Deep Laughter: Allow the laughter to become deep and hearty. It's encouraged to laugh from the belly, allowing the laugh to be as loud and as deep as feels comfortable.
6. Meditative Silence: After a series of laughter exercises, transition into a period of silence. Sit or lie down quietly, allowing the body to relax deeply. Observe the sensations in the body and the calmness of the mind, reflecting on the joy and lightness brought about by laughing.
7. Grounding and Closing: Conclude with a grounding exercise. This could involve some gentle stretching, further deep breathing, or sharing experiences with the group. Reflect on the emotional release and mental clarity experienced during the session.

Regular practice of laughing meditation can improve emotional resilience, reduce stress, and foster a positive outlook on life. It is particularly beneficial for improving social bonds when practiced in groups, enhancing a sense of connection and community. Engaging in laughing meditation can provide a joyful break from the daily routine, promoting health and happiness.

The End

As we reach the end of "Discover Your Meditation," it's important to reflect on the journey you've embarked upon. Exploring different meditation techniques is not just about finding the right practice but also about understanding yourself better and growing in your personal and spiritual life.

We encourage you to reflect on your journey, deepen your practice, and integrate meditation into your daily life for lasting benefits. Embrace the journey with an open heart and mind, and may you find peace and fulfillment in your meditation practice.

Reflecting on Your Journey

Meditation is a deeply personal journey that evolves over time. As you have explored different techniques in this book, you may have discovered methods that resonate with you and others that don't. This is natural and part of the process of finding what works best for you.

Reflect on the following questions to gain insight into your meditation journey:

- Which techniques resonated most with you?

- How did each practice affect your mind, body, and emotions?
- What challenges did you encounter, and how did you overcome them?

Journaling your thoughts and experiences can provide clarity and help you track your progress over time.

Deepening Your Practice

Now that you have a foundation in various meditation techniques, consider these tips for deepening your practice:

- Consistency is Key: Regular practice is crucial for reaping the benefits of meditation. Aim to meditate daily, even if it's just for a few minutes.
- Create a Sacred Space: Designate a specific area in your home for meditation. This can help create a conducive environment and reinforce your commitment to the practice.
- Expand Your Knowledge: Continue learning about meditation through books, workshops, and online resources. Consider attending retreats or joining meditation groups to deepen your understanding and connect with like-minded individuals.
- Listen to Your Body and Mind: Pay attention to how different practices affect you. Adjust your

meditation routine based on your needs and what feels right for you at any given time.

- Incorporate Mindfulness into Daily Life: Practice mindfulness throughout your day by being present in each moment. Whether you're eating, walking, or working, bring the same awareness and presence you cultivate in meditation to your everyday activities.

Integrating Meditation into Your Life

Integrating meditation into your daily life can have profound and lasting benefits. Here are some practical ways to incorporate meditation and mindfulness into your routine:

- Morning Meditation: Start your day with a short meditation session to set a positive tone for the day ahead. Even five to ten minutes of meditation can help you begin your day with clarity and focus.

- Mindful Breaks: Take mindful breaks throughout the day. Pause for a few moments to take deep breaths and center yourself. This can help reduce stress and increase productivity.

- Evening Reflection: End your day with a meditation session or a reflection practice. This can help you unwind, reflect on your day, and promote restful sleep.

- Mindful Activities: Engage in activities mindfully, such as mindful eating, walking, or listening. Focus fully on the activity at hand, bringing your full attention to each moment.

Continuing Your Growth

Meditation is a lifelong journey that evolves as you grow and change. Here are some final thoughts to support your ongoing practice:

- Stay Open and Curious: Remain open to new experiences and techniques. As you grow, your meditation practice may change, and that's perfectly natural.

- Be Kind to Yourself: Meditation is a practice of self-care and self-discovery. Be patient and kind to yourself, especially on challenging days.

- Celebrate Your Progress: Acknowledge and celebrate your progress, no matter how small. Every step on your meditation journey is valuable.

"Discover Your Meditation" has endeavored to provide you with a toolkit of meditation techniques to explore and integrate into your life. Remember that the journey is as important as the destination. By continuing to practice and stay mindful, you will cultivate a deeper sense of peace, clarity, and well-being.

May you continue to grow, discover, and find joy in your practice.

Happy meditating.

Copyright

Cataloging-in-Publication Data
Names: Pathak, Nilam -author. Sharma, Anshuman -author.
Title: Discover Your Meditation / by Nilam Pathak, Anshuman Sharma.
Includes bibliographical references and index.

About Authors

Nilam Pathak

worked with global organizations and institutions to realize the potential of corporate employees, students and masses. She believes in the power of Personality Development and Communication Skills to empower the vulnerable.

She has trained professionals and trainers of various domains and nations. She is an internationally published author of eight books.

Anshuman Sharma

Anshuman is an author and knowledge creator who has transformed the lives and work of people from every continent. His groundbreaking ideas in Thinking, Communication, Personality and Storytelling are revolutionary, simple, and effective.

His belief in simplicity has created powerful solutions that can be used by everyone effortlessly.

www.ingramcontent.com/pod-product-compliance
Lightning Source LLC
Chambersburg PA
CBHW051308250726
48656CB00004B/1536

* 9 7 9 8 3 2 7 8 3 5 0 6 1 *